Rotten Hobby

A True Story of the Unspoken Epidemic Sweeping America

By Jeremy W. Scott
with Daen Scott APRN, FNP-BC, CDE

ROTTEN HOBBY: A TRUE STORY OF THE
UNSPOKEN EPIDEMIC SWEEPING AMERICA
Copyright © 2017 by Jeremy W. Scott

ISBN-13: 978-0692829738
ISBN-10: 0692829733

All scripture quotations are from the *New Revised Standard Version Bible,* copyright 1989, Division of Christian Education of the National Council of the Churches of Christ in the United States of America. All rights reserved.

Fall of Man by Titian (Tiziano Vecellio) (c.1488-1576). Circa 1550. Public domain image from:
https://commons.wikimedia.org/wiki/File:Tizian_091.jpg

For my grandfather, Marshall

Table of Contents

1. The Diagnosis

About one in ten Americans has diabetes, and I am one of them. And, no, I don't look like Wilford Brimley. Not yet anyway. Most of us look like normal people. Meet us on the street and you'd never know we were different from anybody else until you invite us to get donuts. Then, perhaps, we will let you in on our secret.

Most people with diabetes, myself included, don't like talking about it. We don't really want sympathy and we don't want to be treated differently. We look normal and we do all we can to act normal. But sometimes that can be very, very, hard.

Because, the honest truth is this: Having diabetes sucks.

I don't mean the "I had a bad day and my boss yelled at me" kind of sucks. Not a temporary "if I put on a fake smile and get through it now, tomorrow will be better," kind of sucks. I mean a chronic, every day, "I am *never* getting away from this" kind of sucks. If you have had diabetes for a while, you know what I am talking about. If you are reading this because someone you care about has diabetes, this is the first thing they want you to understand. They don't want your pity, but they do need you to know that what they deal with is hard and they never get to take a vacation from it.

My wife, who is awesome in so many ways, is a health-care provider who works in endocrinology. My diabetes pals know what that word means. If you don't, consider that a blessing. Every day she works with patients who have diabetes and, as a specialist, she doesn't work with your average people; she gets the tough cases. The "easy answers don't work so we're going to need to get creative" type cases. Did I mention she's awesome?

In dealing with these folks, she has developed a standard speech she gives, and it starts like this: "Diabetes is the hobby nobody wants." Oh, how true. A good hobby will captivate your attention and time. You'll read books about it, schedule time for it, and generally integrate it into your life in a prominent way. Diabetes is like that, except instead of being an activity you enjoy doing like sports, cooking, or carpentry, it is activities you generally don't want to do. Like stabbing your finger multiple times a day or skipping the cake at the company party and having everyone look at you funny. After all, who doesn't want cake!?

Diabetes truly is a rotten hobby. Worse yet, it is one you get assigned by fate and have little choice in. Like the universe just declared: You will be a Green Bay Packers fan, but you don't live in the Midwest and you don't like cheese! Though, that might be worse, now that I think about it.

All of this is to say: Having diabetes sucks and we need to get that out in the open from the beginning. At no time in the following pages will I offer you any quick fixes or magic solutions. If you want snake oil, check the Internet and you'll find no end of rarified potions to cure your diabetes and regrow your hair to boot. All from reputable places like inner Mongolia and former Eastern Bloc countries. 'Cause, you know, the FDA is keeping all the good shit secret!

This project is different. I want to tell you my story because the more I talk to other people with diabetes, the more I find we have in common. We struggle with guilt and shame. We move through the spectrum of resistance to acceptance and back again constantly. We all hit the "screw it" wall at least once and go on a bender of potato chips and MoonPies. And, most importantly, we all go through this and almost never tell anybody. We struggle and nobody knows, and that is not okay.

So this is my story, or part of it, at least. Some of it may be your story, too. If so, I want you to know one thing most of all: You are not alone.

When you are in your twenties, you think your twenties are pretty great. Later, I would discover what we all do—that your twenties are overrated. But when I was twenty-four, I was having a pretty good time. I had graduated college and had a great job as a software engineer. For the first time in my life I was making good money and, thanks to the insane borrowing practices that would destroy our economy a few years later, I was a homeowner! My wife and I had just gotten married and moved to Albuquerque to start a passionate love affair with green chilies.

I had a job where I traveled constantly. Like, forty-five weeks a year constantly. This meant there were plenty of airline miles and hotel points to take good vacations, and quarterly bonuses sufficient to pay my wife's tuition as she started her undergraduate degree over again (long story).

We were enjoying life.

While I was excited that our newfound financial health allowed us to do things like buy cars and TVs, my wife was excited by something else. She pointed out that we now had real health insurance, and she made us appointments to get physicals. I always thought physicals were for preteens and old people, but I went along. This is why married men live longer, by the way.

I wasn't super excited about going to the doctor. I knew he would tell me I was overweight and would probably want to either put something into my body or take something out, which would involve needles. I hate needles. To this day I cannot look at them. But I love my wife, so I went. No needles this time, but I did get to pee in a cup. Just know—for overweight people this can be a little more challenging than for all you skinny folk.

After we left, I didn't think much about it until a phone call came a couple days later. They wanted me to come back so they could draw some blood and check something called my "fasting blood glucose" and "A1c." What I didn't know at the time was that my urine test came back with too much sugar in it.

You see, if the level of sugar in your blood is too high, your kidneys try to help you out. They let out some sugar and send it off downstream, if you catch my meaning. In fact, not so long ago, before we had all the fancy lab equipment, a doctor would diagnose diabetes by tasting a patient's pee to see if it was sweet. If you are reading this while eating or drinking, I apologize.

Anyway, it took them three tries to find a vein and get the blood that they wanted, which is not a record for me since then. As soon as it was over, I hopped on a plane to Kansas City and my wife went to class. A couple days later we got the second phone call. My fasting blood glucose was over 300 and my A1c was 13 percent. All the people reading this who have diabetes just cringed. For those of you not in the know, that is bad. Like, really bad. The doctor phoned in a prescription for some drugs and scheduled a follow-up.

Like it or not, my life was changing forever.

I grew up on after-school specials that taught me about the things that could ruin your life from an early age. I learned to just say no to drugs, to not impregnate my girlfriend, to not drop out of school. Nowhere in any *The More You Know* segment did A1c's come up.

In a normal person, fasting blood glucose should be under 100 and A1c under 6 percent. The fasting blood glucose measures how much sugar is in your blood at that moment. You are supposed to be fasting, meaning nothing to eat or drink for twelve hours prior, so that your morning Frosted Flakes don't skew the test. Your blood sugar level will naturally fluctuate throughout the day. Eat that office birthday cake and your level will go up. Skip lunch and in the afternoon it may go low, making you feel tired. So the fasting test levels the playing field. Ever wonder why there is a long line of people to get blood drawn first thing in the morning? This is why. Fasting is best done while sleeping.

Too much sugar in blood is the big diabetes issue. It is the thing that will mess you up long term. The A1c test is designed to estimate your average blood sugar level over the past couple months. This lets you know if you are consistently higher or lower than normal. It does this by seeing how many of your red blood cells are coated with sugar. Or, and I am not making this up, how many are *caramelized*. I cannot help but imagine my blood cells wrapped in cellophane, being sold by the pound. That might just be me.

So my fasting blood glucose sucked and my average sucked, meaning, in general, my sugar level sucked. This is a big deal.

Day to day most people with diabetes seem fine. You don't typically notice the fact that your blood sugar is high. You may feel a little off or your joints may hurt a little, but there is nothing to say for sure that it is related to your blood sugar. Could be you just got a bad night's sleep.

Diabetes is not the kind of condition where things happen quickly or suddenly; it is more insidious than that. Things happen over time— months and years. Besides being overweight, at twenty-four I felt pretty good, despite the fact that I had likely been running around with elevated blood sugar levels for a couple of years at the least. So you might be asking, what's the big deal? Well, let me tell you.

Too much sugar in your blood can mess up almost every system in your body. Over time, the vessels that carry your blood can start to harden and your smaller capillaries (very small blood vessels) can be damaged. These capillaries are important, especially in places like your eyes. On the backs of your eyeballs are lots of very small capillaries and if these are damaged they can start to leak. This is called diabetic retinopathy, and it can make you go blind. Like, for real blind. In fact, eye doctors first notice many new cases of diabetes when they start to see bleeding on the back of the eye.

Now, your body needs the sugar that is in your blood. It is literally what all your cells runs on. All the food you spend hours combining into a delicious form, when you eat it, gets immediately broken down into various components, with sugar being a primary one. Every cell needs some sugar to function. It is estimated that an average adult brain uses 250 M&M's worth of sugar every day. You are candy powered!

To use that sugar, your body creates a hormone called insulin in your pancreas. Insulin is like a hall monitor for your body as it regulates how much sugar your cells can take in. Otherwise they would just gorge themselves when your blood sugar is high and starve when it is not. Your body needs to keep some sugar in your blood to even things out and keep the feast/famine cycle from hurting you. But if your levels are already high for other reasons, your pancreas will overproduce insulin to try to get it down, and this could damage it. Also, your cells can start to get resistant to the insulin, leaving more sugar in your blood than is good for you and harming those blood vessels. Think of having high blood sugar like a high school where all the kids are in the hallways instead of in class. Nothing useful gets done and stuff gets broken.

Diabetes is, at the end of the day, a cardiovascular issue. It can lead to poor circulation, nerve damage, and heart attacks. People with diabetes must regularly check their feet for nicks or cuts because poor circulation and numbness can mean small wounds can be overlooked and are prone to infection. As a bonus, blood that is full of sugar doesn't fight off infections well. This is why you hear of people losing feet, legs, and other extremities to diabetes. They get infected and it goes unnoticed for too long.

So day to day you feel, look, and act normal. Yet at the same time, your body is slowly being eroded from the inside out, setting up potentially massive complications down the road. We are frogs in a pot of water and the temperature is slooooowly increasing.

This is the world I entered at age twenty-four when I was supposed to be occupied with starting a career and a family. Needless to say, I was not happy about it.

Diabetes is not just a diagnosis; it is a whole new lifestyle. If you are going to keep the worst of the potential complications at bay, you have to learn a whole new way of relating to food and your environment. Sure, I got a prescription for some pills (hands up for Metformin!), but that was just the start. When I was diagnosed, it felt like I became the center of a messed-up universe. I was on the road so my wife waited a couple of days to pick up my prescription. This didn't go over well with our new doctor and my wife got a phone call informing her we needed to take this seriously and start my new medication quickly. Next came the classes with a nutritionist to tell me how I was eating wrong and diabetes educators to tell me how my body was trying to pickle itself. Really uplifting stuff! Everything felt so urgent and all I heard were dire predictions of terrible things to come. It took me months to figure out that I needed to not give in to the panic growing inside of me but instead work things one step at a time. If you are newly diagnosed I feel for you. Breathe; it will be okay.

My meeting with the nutritionist was a group class, run by a former hippie. She started by asking us to write down what we ate in a normal day. I don't say this lightly, because I am certain of very little in life, but I am certain of this: all of us lied. As she reviewed our lists she asked each of us in turn if we felt satisfied by the amount of food we wrote down? Of course, we all answered yes, which was so very untrue, and she replied with a knowing, "Uh-huh." I wish I still had a copy of mine. I am sure vegetables featured more prominently on the list than in reality, meaning they were actually on the list. One guy went off about how if he was feeling hungry he would just steam up some broccoli for a snack. Sure, man, right. That is why we're all here, too much broccoli.

I was assigned a diet that allowed up to sixty grams of carbohydrates per meal, no snacks, and no soda or juice. We reviewed how nutrition labels worked and that you could subtract dietary fiber from the total carbs listed. Score! It was actually a useful experience and it helped me become aware that I honestly had no clue about what I was eating on a regular basis even though I thought I did. I know many people brush off these opportunities, figuring they already know what they need to know. Don't be one of those people.

As helpful as the food information was, something else the nutritionist said stuck with me: "You didn't break yourself." She wanted us to know that we weren't failures, and we weren't there because we did something wrong or were bad people. This was good to hear, even though at the time I was too caught up in my new day-to-day reality that I hadn't had a chance to reflect on why or how I had gotten there. That would come later.

On the whole, I agree with her reassurance from years ago. Having diabetes doesn't mean you are a failure or a bad person. Feeling guilty or ashamed does you no good at all. Diabetes runs in families, and your genes can make you more or less at risk for developing it. It is important to realize diabetes also comes in different forms.

I have type 2 diabetes, and up to this point that is what I have been talking about. Type 2 used to be called adult-onset diabetes. The other, type 1, was called juvenile diabetes. Types 1 and 2 are different based on what causes them. Type 2 happens when your cells become resistant to the insulin in your body, leaving more sugar in your blood. Type 1 happens when your body's immune system damages part of your pancreas, where insulin is made, and thus limits your body's ability to make its own insulin. Again, leaving too much sugar in your blood. Today we can make insulin that can be injected to supplement for a type 1's low production.

Just a few decades ago that was not true, and being diagnosed type 1 was basically a diagnosis for an early death. Even after insulin became available, there were problems in knowing how much to take. Remember, you don't normally feel your blood sugar being too high, but you can certainly feel it when it is too low. So most people favored being slightly higher than risk going low. Today, we have small machines you can carry with you that can tell you what your blood sugar level is in a matter of seconds. This has greatly improved the quality and span of life for type 1s.

There was a time when type 2 diabetes was properly called adult onset because only older adults got it. It takes time for chronically high blood sugar levels to cause your body to become resistant to insulin. In fact, it used to take decades. My grandfather was diagnosed with type 2 in his fifties, which is pretty common, with one in four older adults being diagnosed. However, back in the 1990s, something new started to happen. Children and teens started to pop up all over the United States with type 2 diabetes. Our country that craves things ever faster and cheaper had figured out how to accelerate chronic diseases. Go America!

So yes, I am predisposed to diabetes by my grandfather and would have at some point likely developed the condition. So yes, this is not my fault. That said, I did start asking myself why I was diagnosed at twenty-four and my grandfather got a free pass 'til his mid-fifties. The truth is that while the "if I were to ever get diabetes" question was likely not up to me, the "when would I develop it" question was being informed by my lifestyle. Drive around long enough on an underinflated tire and you will have a blowout. Drag race with it and it will happen a great deal sooner.

Every person with diabetes I know eventually comes to this point. They realize they ultimately had no choice in the matter, but at the same time they sort of did. And this, my friends, is a particularly un-fun place to be.

In the months that followed my diagnosis I was still traveling most weeks. I had moved from a project based out of Kansas City (great barbeque) to one right across the George Washington Bridge from Manhattan (great everything). We had a $125-a-day food reimbursement and more topflight restaurant choices than this raised-in-rural-eastern-Montana boy could contemplate.

On paper, sixty grams of carbs per meal should be plenty. In practice, it felt woefully inadequate. Most restaurant menus didn't list nutrition information, and Steve Jobs had not yet given the world a proper smartphone. So I was left to estimate, something I got good at doing. Though, let's be honest, what I got good at was underestimating.

Things at home weren't all that much better. I was the cook in the house (still am), and I had inherited mostly pasta-dish recipes from my mother. Not to mention, even when I was home we still ate out constantly thanks to my wife and my crazy schedules. Non-diet soda was banned from the house but my wife insisted on keeping real juice around, over my protests. I almost never poured a glass, but many servings were ingested straight from the container. A note to all wives out there: husbands do this. Though we try to do it when you aren't looking, which I think is an important gesture.

When you are diagnosed with either type of diabetes, you get new equipment to carry with you: a blood glucose meter. Someone teaches you how to use the lancet (a nice word for something you stab yourself with) to extract a small amount of blood from your finger. This blood then goes on a strip placed in the small device that a few moments later gives you a report about your value as a human being and your moral failure rating for the day. Or, at least, that is how it feels. What it really tells you is your blood glucose level.

One of the most common times to test is first thing in the morning, for the same reason they did a fasting blood glucose test on me when I was being diagnosed. Which means your day, every day, begins with this. The issue is, your test result can only be one of two things: normal or bad. So at best you are simply the same as everyone else. At worst, you are not as good as everyone else. For a time I also was weighing myself, since having diabetes is correlated with being overweight. But I had to stop doing that or risk my wife taking my shoelaces away for fear I might do something rash.

Most of us already live in a world that offers far too many ways to compare ourselves to others via how much money we make, the car we drive, or the level of education we've received. Having diabetes only adds new ways to measure yourself against that most horrible of standards, *normal people*. I have never been one to worry much about what normal people do, but suddenly I was thrust into a world where that seemed to be all that mattered.

To be fair, it is not like this all the time. Relatively quickly it becomes routine. You get up, prick your finger, write down the number then go take a shower. You pass on all the optional desserts (some just aren't optional) and pretend to like diet soda until you actually do. With luck you can stretch this time of normalness for weeks or months. On the whole, I would say my life has been more times like this than not, which is good. But since diabetes never really goes away, it is always lurking in the background, and it will eventually find a way to break through your veil of normalcy.

While working on that project right off Manhattan, our team discovered a local Italian restaurant which became the place we could all agree on. At least once a week we would go there and indulge. This particular place didn't serve wine or beer itself, but you could bring your own. Conveniently there was a liquor store right next door. So our first stop was there, then off for some of the finest red sauce I have had before or since.

One particular Wednesday night, we forwent the wine and bought a bottle of vodka instead. It barely survived until the main course arrived and we were all grateful the hotel shuttle would be picking us up and nobody needed to drive. To be sure, there were more nights of excess drinking in those days than is advisable. This is what happens when you are a team made up almost entirely of people who only recently were fully released into adulthood.

That night I enjoyed my pasta and decided to also enjoy some dessert. This was not a common part of our meals together and I soon discovered I was the only one to order something. As we waited for it to arrive, and folks pondered the empty vodka bottle, one colleague chimed in, "I thought you weren't supposed to have things like that?"

"Things like what?" I replied.

"Like what you ordered. The dessert."

"No, probably not, but it won't kill me."

At this point, with nothing else to do, another inquired, "Why can't you have it?"

"He's got diabetes!" the first helpfully replied.

Things devolved from there and I found myself giving a basic primer on my condition to a group of mostly inebriated engineers who in that moment possessed the emotional intelligence of your average middle schooler.

"So why are you having that?" each asked in their own only mildly differentiated way. And, of course, I didn't really have an answer. The truth is people aren't logical, and we don't really make decisions based on what's best for us long term. That is why we have to be bribed into saving for retirement through matching 401ks and we have gym memberships we don't use. In the abstract, as an idea, I knew dessert was a poor life choice, but in the moment I just wanted some damned crème brûlée!

Not only was my secret out, I now had the joy of welcoming a dozen new people to my own personal cadre of food police. Even if they never said anything again, I would feel like every sandwich I ate in front of them was being judged. And even if they weren't actually doing that, I would be. To an outsider, the whole incident would look very tame. I doubt anyone overhearing the conversation would have thought much of it. Yet, of the dozens of times we gathered around a table at that restaurant, this is the only one I remember so vividly. Looking back, I must confess there is no evidence that any of them treated me any differently after, but at the time I felt awful, like a failure, and left the dessert mostly unfinished. We could not get back to the hotel fast enough.

For a time, normalcy was broken and I was reminded that I was different. It would return, routine would return, and life would go on. But the experience and the emotions that went with it are something I can always relive, even when I don't want to.

In this way, having diabetes is like any other chronic condition. It is always there. Most of the time you just ignore it, work around it, and try not to give it any more energy or thought than you have to. Sometimes, though, it comes front and center into your life uninvited and you have no choice but to deal with it. What might seem like a minor thing to those not currently inside your brain with you is experienced as a big deal to you and can set off a chain reaction of unhealthy responses.

Truly, having diabetes sucks. Sometimes just a little, and at random intervals a lot. So you adjust, adapt, and deal with it. Because the other thing I would learn shortly after my diagnosis is that I am stronger than it is. And so are you.

2. The Stacked Deck

A diagnosis of any type of diabetes comes with several prescriptions. Some of them are for pills, which help but don't cure. Most are for learning things. Visits to nutritionists and diabetes educators help you understand what is going on in your body and why you need to eat and act differently. I know few people who get excited about these visits, but they are actually quite important.

People newly diagnosed with diabetes go through a sort of discovery process. You take your home blood glucose meter and go on a scavenger hunt to figure out what foods will up your blood sugar count the most. The process is pretty straightforward. You eat a reasonable portion of whatever you're wondering about, drink plenty of water, then wait two hours without eating anything. Then you prick your finger and test your level. In no time you learn what's a good two-hour reading and what's a bad one. I tended to lump things into one of a few categories. Nobody told me to do this, but I am an engineer by training and believe the whole world should be put into categories. It is what we do.

Here are mine:

1. Generally OK. Things made up of mostly protein like meat and nuts and something called *vegetables* which I was just learning about.

2. Once(ish) a Day. More carb-heavy things like cereal, thick sandwich bread, and most fruit.

3. Once a Week. All my mother's pasta dishes.

4. In Case of Emergency. Reserved for truly horrible days or family holiday meals which all seem designed to kill people with diabetes.

5. Last meal on Earth. A regular Coke and a box of Girl Scout cookies.

An important note: This only has to do with blood sugar, not anything else. You cannot live off meat and nuts. Other complications will quickly set in if you try. No reason to avoid a diabetic heart attack by having a cholesterol-induced one. I have been told you can live off of vegetables and fruit, I believe these people are called vegetarians, but I don't think I will be walking that road anytime soon.

As I continued my journey of food discovery, I became more and more disgusted with what I found. Every item in the grocery store that is not fresh fruit, vegetables, or meat has a standard nutrition label on it. We've all seen them, and you were perhaps even taught how to read them in school. However, I have never in my entire life seen anyone at the grocery store actually pick up a package and check the label. All the information is there but we never read it.

There is this myth that is widely told in various forms that we want to believe is true. It goes something like this. *People want to be well informed, and if they are well informed they will make good and healthy choices.* Oh, how we wish this were true. We wish it so much we make public-policy decisions based on it. For evidence, look no further than any package of cigarettes.

For decades, cigarettes, cigars, and smokeless tobacco products have been more than happy to inform us that using these products will kill you. Or, if not kill you, make truly awful things happen to you. Yet, despite doing this for longer than I have been alive, many people still smoke. True, the rate is coming down, but only very slowly. It took over forty years to cut the smoking rate in the US in half. Forty years!

So if the strategy of *an informed consumer is a healthy consumer* takes decades to make real change when the math is DOING THIS = DEATH!, how much harder is it when the math is DOING THIS + LOTS OF TIME = POSSIBLE HEALTH ISSUES (MAYBE)?

Coca-Cola kicked off the diet soda craze in 1963 with Tab. Some of you will remember its bright-pink can and groovy font. Because, you know, it was for the ladies. At this time the diabetes rate in the US was right at 1 percent according to the Centers for Disease Control, and it had been at about this level for as long as they had been tracking it. What started with Tab blossomed into a whole diet-food movement that would lead to prepackaged meals, dieting cookbooks, and an ever-increasing cadre of chemical sugar substitutes.

Before the mid-sixties food was just, well, food. You went to the store to buy ingredients to take home and prepare food. Frozen dinners were just starting to become a thing, as most cooking was still done at home, not in some far-off factory.

By the way, I don't mean to sound nostalgic about this time. Valium-popping stay-at-home moms were all too common a thing as women bore too much of the burden of keeping the nuclear family together. The rampant sexism and racism of this age is not something to aspire to return to. In fact, when convenient, heat-and-eat, processed food came on the market it was seen as a tool to liberate women from the kitchen. Dinner did not have to take an hour to prepare; it could be minutes! Add the newly invented microwave to the mix and America's eating habits changed in a flash. This revolution was almost complete by the time I entered the scene in the late seventies. I grew up in a home that always had a microwave and a freezer full of readymade food-like products wrapped in plastic. Most conveniently delivered to our home by the Schwan's Man.

For basically forever, if you wanted something high in fat or sugar to eat, it took a long time to prepare. Birthday cake is a thing because, before the factory-food revolution, cakes were a pain in the butt to make. Honestly, go bake a cake, not from a box but ingredient by ingredient, and then whip up your own icing from scratch. My wife does this from time to time and it takes forever! Or, bake a pie. Like, a real pie, with fresh filling and homemade crust. We only do these things on birthdays or holidays because that is the only time we can justify the effort. So, not so long ago, the only time you had access to these types of foods was a handful of days a year.

Today, a dollar will buy you an individually wrapped, ready-to-eat Hostess Fruit Pie any time you desire. Complete with sixty-eight grams of sugar! This is unprecedented in the entire history of humanity. So it should surprise no one that the rates of diabetes and obesity grow at a steady pace along with the increasing adoption of the processed food that makes it oh so easy to consume far more sugar and fat than you should.

The game *is* rigged and the deck *is* stacked against you.

Perhaps the best way to understand this is through the story of one of the greatest love affairs of my life. My love for soda. Coke to be specific. It was, for me, the standard beverage of my life. Go out to eat, order a Coke. At the cafeteria in college, drink Coke. Go to the fridge, grab a Coke. Pepsi is a poor substitute, only to be drunk in an emergency. Like, when the restaurant doesn't have Coke. It is not like I was going to drink water, after all.

In the summer of 1999, a year before my diagnosis, I was asked by the company I was working for to go to Germany for a few months to work on a project there. I was excited to go as I had not been out of the country since I was very little and I was ready for some adventure. I didn't think much about the fact that I spoke no German, figuring I would be spending most of my time with my computer, writing and debugging code. That part turned out to be true. What I did not count on was that Germany had a very different relationship with food than I did. In the part of the country I was in, people still shopped at grocery stores for ingredients. Rather small stores at that. Bread was bought at a different store (the *Konditorei*) and fresh meat at yet another store. I also quickly noticed that my colleagues packed lunches to work, something I had stopped doing in about seventh grade. It was a whole different world.

By month two of being there, the cultural isolation was getting to me and I became increasingly grateful for the one outpost of

American cultural superiority to be had in my German lake town: McDonald's. It was over two miles from my apartment and several times a week I walked there. I would order a Number One (*Nummer Eins*) because a Big Mac is a Big Mac no matter where in the world you are. There was no supersize to be had, so you got the same sized drink everyone got. I think it was around sixteen ounces. It was here, with my ridiculously undersized soda, that I learned there was something wrong with German people. Sure, you could get a beer at McDonald's, but I didn't want that. What I wanted was an ice-cold, refreshing, and well-sized Coke. Apparently this was too much to ask for.

First, German McDonald's serves their soda with no lid or straw and with about a half dozen small ice cubes floating at the top. So, ice cold is out. Second, the size was suitable for a Happy Meal but not for an adult. Finally, and most importantly, if you finished it they expected you to buy another one. No free refills! What the hell is wrong with this country?

One day I convinced my coworkers to put aside their sack lunches full of homemade goodness and come with me to get Big Macs at America Land. During the meal, I ranted just a little about their weird soda practices. When I got to the part about the free refill the conversation just stopped. For a time I thought we were having a translation issue. I still spoke very little German and their English was passable but not fluent. So I slowed down and tried to explain the concept a few different ways, including miming it out. As it happens, the words were not the problem; they understood those. What they didn't understand was why anyone would want more soda. For them, the measly serving they have been conditioned to see as normal was sufficient. My respect for them obviously dropped dramatically.

A few months after I returned, one of my German coworkers came to our office in the US and stayed in my spare room for a while. Being the hospitable person I am, I of course took him to the McDonald's across the street. During our lunch, Big Macs, he suddenly started laughing. He had just noticed the soda fountain was out where customers could serve themselves and they were happily getting refill after refill. He then told me he thought I was kidding when I went on that rant back in Germany, and he needed to come back with his camera and get a picture. "Nobody will believe me back home," he said.

Germans are weird.

To be fair, Germans are not immune to the diabetes epidemic, as their rates increase along with ours. Since my visit many years ago, Germany has developed one of the worst rates in Europe. And it's not just Germany; rates are increasing everywhere, with the worldwide rate doubling in the last twenty-five years.

I am also not scapegoating soda as the main issue, but I do strongly believe it is part of the equation. To illustrate that, another story.

New Coke is a punch line for those who happened to live through this dark period in soda history. For those ignorant of this Reagan-era insanity, let me explain. In 1985, Coca-Cola did the unthinkable and changed the flavor of its flagship product. The reason given at the time was that they wanted to reformulate the taste to reach a younger audience. Pepsi was in full swing with its head-to-head "Pepsi Challenge," and New Coke was purported to be Coke fighting back.

Despite what their advertising might try to convince you of, Coke as a company is not really about world peace or turning mean football players nice. It is a company, and like all other companies, its purpose is to make money. Coca-Cola sells soda, and sells more regular Coke than anything else. To make more profit, meaning income minus expenses, you either have to increase income or lower expenses. That is just basic economics. When New Coke was rolled out, it was pitched as an attempt to increase income when, in reality, it was actually about lowering expenses. Never heard this part of the story? No surprise. In 1985, with no internet, YouTube, or Drudge Report to distribute crazy conspiracies, we basically had to take what companies told us at face value.

When you sell sugary beverages for a living, your biggest expense is, no surprise, sugar. Up 'til New Coke came to market, Coke was sweetened with real sugar like you buy in the store. Problem is, real sugar can be expensive. Most domestic sugar comes from sugar beets grown in the northern part of the country. Cane sugar comes from warmer climates like Brazil and other parts of South America. Cane sugar has tariffs on it, making it expensive to import. Sugar beets only grow in certain areas and take a lot of land and time to develop. Sugar, the real thing Coke sells, is also its most expensive ingredient.

However, America does grow a whole bunch of something else: corn! In the second half of the twentieth century, food scientists figured out how to make a very sweet yet inexpensive product, called high-fructose corn syrup, that could be used as an almost direct replacement for natural sugar. This highly processed ingredient was quickly marketed to all sorts of customers, including soda makers.

It takes little to no imagination to picture what transpired in the Coca-Cola boardroom in the early eighties. They wanted to switch sweeteners so they could save a ton of cash, and, since nutrition and ingredient label laws would not exist 'til 1990, the switch would not show up on the can's nonexistent ingredient list. The only challenge was that it would taste just a little different and, if people started to ask why, they'd have to confess they were switching to a lower-cost ingredient, which would look bad. In this light, the choice becomes obvious—tweak the taste at the same time and nobody would be the wiser. My guess is the genius who came up with this got a mighty fat bonus.

Most of us know where the story goes: New Coke is a flop and, within the year, Coke Classic comes out and is advertised as going back to the original taste. However, it didn't, not really. They might have gone back to the original recipe for most things but they kept the new sweetener. Forever after, Coke would be made with high-fructose corn syrup in the US, while real sugar would continue to be the main ingredient elsewhere.

Sugar, like you buy in the store, is actually made up of a 50/50 mix of two different types of sugar at the molecular level: fructose and glucose. They look and taste similar and contain a similar number of calories, but your body processes them differently. A study was done at Yale University where researchers gave volunteers two different drinks, one sweetened only with fructose and the other only glucose, then they scanned their brains in an MRI machine. What they discovered was that the bodies of those who drank the glucose-based drink responded in a way that would cause their appetites to decrease and lead to a feeling of fullness. Conversely, those who drank the fructose-based drink didn't have the same reaction so didn't get the benefit of reduced appetite and feeling full.

Most high-fructose corn syrup used in food manufacturing today contains a higher percentage of fructose than glucose. So while it is true that high-fructose corn syrup and regular sugar are comparable in terms of calories, they are not the same in how they work in your body. According to studies, eating food made with high-fructose corn syrup leads to you not feeling as full, your body producing less insulin, thus leaving more sugar in your blood, and makes it easier to overeat by not reducing your appetite as much.

All this is important for a couple of reasons. First, for the last few decades of the twentieth century, as obesity rates climbed, fat in food was made to be the main culprit in the American diet. We were told over and over that fat was bad and we needed to reduce it at all costs. In college I worked in the dining hall and once asked the on-staff nutritionist to help me eat better and maybe lose some weight. Later that week she caught me just as I lifted a Rice Krispies Treat from the dessert table. "No problem," she said, "those are fat free." *Fantastic!* I thought in reply, and took two.

Around the country, out went eggs and avocados while food manufacturers rushed to create fat-free or low-fat products. The problem is that fat-free food, especially heavily processed food like you get from a factory, tastes like cardboard. It is truly terrible. So, in order to make it palatable the sweetener industry was more than happy to offer a solution. So the fat was taken out of food and sugar and high-fructose corn syrup came in. This did lead to a small reduction in total calories per serving in some cases, but somehow the epidemic of diabetes and obesity continued. In fact, while the whole diet-food industry flourished, the rates for all sorts of diet-related conditions exploded. So you have to ask yourself, what's going on here? If we spend more money than ever on diet books, diet food, and diet drinks, why is the overall health of the country getting worse and worse? We are obviously doing something wrong, but what?

The honest answer is likely not one reason but several. That is a problem because everyone can just point fingers at everyone else. The reality is that sugar in any form is not healthy for you in the quantities we eat it in today. The addition of cheap high-fructose corn syrup just means it can be put in that many more products. So, if you are a food manufacturer, what are you going to do to make your product more palatable? We now find added sugar or high-fructose corn syrup in tomato sauce, ketchup, salad dressing, barbeque sauce, granola bars, canned fruit, dried fruit, nearly every type of premade beverage, and even several varieties of packaged meat. The more you go looking for sugar, the more you find it. It is everywhere!

So this is the world I started to encounter when I was trying to navigate my way through my new diagnosis. I could hardly believe all the places I found sugar lurking. As I studied the nutrition labels I became painfully aware of how quickly it all added up. As I wrestled with the fact that my eating habits likely accelerated the onset of my condition, I also felt like what I was eating was out of my control. When even hamburger buns get their golden top from added sugar, what are you supposed to do?

This would be the beginning of something I would wrestle with for years to come. Even though I wanted to change how I was eating, I found a dearth of drive-through salad options. I didn't just need to change what I was eating but how and where I was eating. I would have to spend far more time and energy thinking about it than I ever had. The scale of it all felt daunting and regularly came to a head as I scavenged restaurant menus while traveling for work to find *something* I would not feel guilty for eating.

This is the world someone with diabetes lives in. One where it feels like everyone is free to indulge in the free-flowing high-carb lifestyle that permeates the globe. Everyone but you. Because, not only do you have to learn to say yes to the right things, you must learn to say no to the wrong things. You cannot just eat the broccoli and the cake; they won't cancel each other out. It doesn't work that way. Too often you feel like you've said no enough and you just want to go with the flow like everyone else and request the big corner piece of the office birthday cake celebrating what's-her-name. Is that so much to ask? Well, your blood glucose meter will tell you in a couple hours that yes, it was too much. Assuming, of course, you have the courage to check. Most times I didn't.

The world is unfortunately not likely to change anytime soon. The sugar and corn lobbies are as powerful as the oil lobby in Washington and we will be hooked on cheap sweetener far longer than oil at the rate things are currently going. It will take years to unlearn that cutting fat at all costs was the wrong approach and that slow, homemade food is vastly preferable to fast food. It will take me years from this point to adapt my own eating habits, with many pitfalls along the way.

Since diagnosis, my A1c has been as low as 6.5 and as high as 11, despite an ever-changing cocktail of the best the pharmaceutical industry has to offer. I both love and hate the stories I hear about people losing massive amounts of weight and their diabetes with it. "Good for them," is my first reaction, followed quickly by, "I sort of hate you." I have contemplated gastric bypass surgery, which for some has worked wonders. I have given myself deadlines; if I am not doing *this good* by *this time* then we will try something more extreme. At least once I hit that limit and went for it which both helped and did not (more on that in chapter seven).

So here is the real thing. Having diabetes in America today is like playing blackjack against a stacked deck. It really does feel like no matter how hard you try, you are doomed to lose. With the final kicker being, you can't just stop playing.

Leaving the table isn't a choice you can make. You have to play because you have to eat.

3. Fathers and Faith

I need to add a couple new parts of my story here. First, I need to tell you about my dad, and second, I need to tell you about my faith. I recognize we live in a world that wants to have less and less to do with religion or faith. Most people are moving through their daily lives not giving much thought to either. I get that. I also am not going to try to push any agenda besides telling my story. If you are not interested in God, that is fine, but please keep reading. Faith may not be part of your story but it is part of mine.

My parents were married young by today's standards, but not by the standards of their day. My father was in the Navy and my mother stayed home to care for my sister, brother, and me. I am the middle child. My father being in the Navy means I got to be born in Rota, Spain, which is listed on my passport. This one fact causes all sorts of strange looks from customs when I travel internationally, as I could pass for a German long before I could pass for a Spaniard. We left Spain when I was two when my dad was reassigned and I would not leave the country again until that trip to Germany. By the time I was six my father had left the Navy and we were living in Texas, outside Fort Hood, while he worked for a military supply contractor. He was an electrician, maintaining their fleet of Bradley Fighting Vehicles. A couple years ago I saw a movie about all the problems with this rather infamous military boondoggle, but at the time all I knew was that my dad worked on tanks.

When you are a six-year-old boy there is no more impressive job in the universe than working on tanks. Especially when you get to visit and sit in one. And I did!

On a nondescript weekend in early September, a couple of weeks into my second-grade year, I was sleeping in my top bunk with my two-year-old brother below me. Unbeknownst to me, my father left that morning to go fishing with a friend and would not come back. At the age of thirty he accidently drowned and it took authorities several days to recover his body. That morning my mother came in our room and woke us up to tell us the news. For some reason, all I remember thinking was, *Do not cry. Show them how big you are and do not cry.* So I didn't. For years.

My father's death kicked off a whirlwind of activity. The next day, family we only saw maybe once a year were in our house. My aunt, my grandparents, they were all there. I was only slightly aware of all the plans being made around me. My mother hated Texas and had no intention of staying. Her parents lived in Sunnyvale, California, and that was where we would be going, at least for a while.

Up until this I had no reason to think my second-grade year would not be in Texas with my friends, siblings, and both parents. In the end my father had not been gone for two weeks before I found myself in California, enrolled in a new school, back in first grade for reasons I still don't understand, and living with my grandparents by myself for over a month while my mother, brother, and sister packed up the house in Texas. It was easy to surmise I was deemed unhelpful to that effort.

So I went to school, watched TV, and ate graham crackers. Lots of graham crackers. Years later I would learn that my grandparents had no idea how to comfort me so they let me do the one thing I seemed to want to do: eat. When I was finally reunited with my family, my mother didn't immediately recognize me at the airport because of the weight I had gained.

The CDC in their Adverse Childhood Experiences (ACE) study found it was very common for those who are considered obese by medical standards to have experienced some sort of childhood trauma. This could be one or a combination of things, like sexual abuse, loss of a parent, or living with an alcoholic. Food becomes a coping mechanism in places of high stress because, honestly, eating sweet and fatty things makes you feel good. I have no doubt there is more science behind it than that, but I am not sure it is necessary. I have spent most of my life eating and drinking the wrong kinds of food in oversized amounts because I like it and it makes me happy. It is the same reason a smoker looks at a warning on a pack of cigarettes, ignores it, and lights up anyway. They like smoking. It makes them feel good.

I needed to make changes in my eating to avoid the worst of the side effects diabetes has to offer. As I tried to do that I found myself fighting hard with... myself. It is as if part of my brain, deep down in the animal part where we don't process words, only emotion, is fighting with the logical part of my brain, the part where I filed away all my college calculus classes. I know what I am supposed to do, but I don't do it. Or at least I don't do it all the time. I am increasingly convinced that the part of me I am fighting with is that sad, lonely, lost six-year-old boy who is attempting to comfort himself however he can. He is still there, in my head, even after several therapy and counseling sessions in the intervening years.

The truth is that twenty-four-year-old me was doomed almost from the start: born into a world where factory food injects extra sugar into every product, genetically predisposed by some unknown ancestor, and visited at an early age by legitimate tragedy.

Mind you, none of this is me attempting to offer excuses, though I am sometimes sorely tempted to make them. What I am hoping to show is that there are reasons why all of us are who we are. Some of those reasons are under our control and some are not. I have personally found dealing with my diabetes and the associated weight issues more akin to dealing with an addiction than anything else. This might sound like a reach but I don't think it is. My body and brain are conditioned at this point for a certain, albeit unhealthy, relationship with food. My daily routine is built around what I see as normal eating, which includes more drive-through runs than is advisable. The daily habits of my life reinforce how I eat, and those habits are hard to break. Even when I know I shouldn't, even when the logical part of my brain is screaming at me, some days I just leave it on autopilot and do what I've always done.

And here is the real gut punch: Your body will fight back if you try to change too much. In your brain there is a setting for how much your body thinks it should weigh. The thinking part of your brain has nothing to say about where the level is set. If you've spent a good part of your life overweight then your body will adjust to that. If you later start to lose some weight through diet and exercise, you are a hero (legit!), but your body will see it differently. It will fight to keep you from going down too much by lowering your metabolism. Seriously, this is science.

In a rare case of reality TV doing something useful, a study was done with fourteen participants from *The Biggest Loser*. They started the show at an average weight of 328 pounds and during the show's run got down to an average of about 200 pounds. However, after all the cameras, personal trainers, and other support left, all but one—one!!—regained nearly everything they had lost. Why? Well, the study also found that despite all the dieting and exercise, their metabolisms had actually slowed down by 27 percent. Meaning, their bodies were using fewer calories in a typical day and storing more in fat. Which is the exact opposite of what you want if you want to lose weight. Their own bodies lowered their metabolism to keep them at the higher weight it was used to.

I am sure there is some evolutionary imperative why our bodies work this way, but to me it is a Darwinian bitch slap of epic proportions. Certain drugs are so powerfully addictive because your brain starts to crave them after exposure and it will do all it can to not allow you to function normally without them. Your brain will change how your body works so that it won't function correctly without the drugs. Turns out your brain does the same thing for food. It will do all it can to keep you from using all the energy you can from what you eat and instead store it as fat.

This is why, for me, dealing with all the interconnected issues of weight, eating, blood sugar, etc. seems a whole lot more like overcoming an addiction than any watered-down "lifestyle choice" language. Drinking Pepsi or wearing ironic eyeglasses is a lifestyle choice; this feels like war.

At this point I am even bumming myself out.

In the book *The Art of War*, Sun Tzu says you must know your enemy. Well, I was learning mine. I had to for one obvious reason. While you can live without drinking alcohol, smoking, or gambling, you cannot live without eating. So you must continue to stay at the table and play against the stacked deck in more ways than you ever realized. My education would take years and continues even now.

At age twenty-six it became clear to me that another transition was on the horizon. The start-up company I had worked for had sold itself for pennies and my once-vaunted private stock didn't amount to enough for a down payment on a new car let alone anything more. Spending a year on a beach somewhere was out. It was also clear that the company that bought us was not any better run than we were, which is to say, not well at all. So I started to look for a new opportunity that might also let me be at home more.

I found a new job at a company with an office only a mile or so from my house in Albuquerque. I could even walk if I wanted, which was admittedly rare. I liked the work, and the regular 8-to-5 hours combined with being home each night felt amazing. I had free time for the first time in my adult life. Too bad I had no idea what to do with it.

There aren't too many hobbies that you can practice from a hotel room five nights a week. Especially in the days before universal free Wi-Fi. That part of my life was not well developed when I suddenly found myself with loads of night and weekend time. Add to that, my wife was often busy on those nights and weekends working live theater shows as she finished her theater degree.

I was listless and needed something more to do. I am not sure why I thought going to church might help but that is what I did. We didn't really go to church a lot growing up though I did participate in youth group and I loved church summer camp. At camp I felt like I could really be myself. To this day those experiences still form me. I suppose at twenty-six I hoped church would be a little like those experiences.

I started to attend the early service at one of the large United Methodist congregations in town. It was mostly an older crowd but that meant they sang the songs I remembered from childhood, so that worked. I went off and on for several months while my wife stayed home and slept in. She was a person of no real religious preference at this point, what would later be termed a "none." As in, *none of the above* for religious preference on surveys. She was not against me going to church but didn't feel it necessary to go herself.

I found some things attending church that I needed. First, I found something to do. I started to work with the youth group since that was all I really knew of church. Which, while fun, was also a bit full of drama since young people are also a bit full of drama. More importantly I also found a way to understand myself better through the idea of brokenness. I had always felt that my life was not quite right. Somehow others seemed to have it more together than I did. They seemed more confident and self-aware than I was. I would look at the lives of others and think they just seemed more complete than mine. So the concept of being broken spoke to me powerfully.

Brokenness is part of the human condition, something we are born with. We don't arrive on Earth fully formed but instead more like raw clay ready to be shaped by the place, time, and family we are born into. Sure, we have some basic structures in our nature, but it is how we are nurtured (or not) in life that will give us our form. Brokenness is the realization that no matter how perfect things may seem on the outside, there are always cracks and imperfections where things didn't go totally to plan. Not only that, but everyone has them and they are normal. Embracing brokenness means not hiding the cracks but instead recognizing they are part of what makes you, you. The broken parts can actually add beauty and depth if we can learn to see them differently. Our brokenness gives us our character.

At church, I learned not to run from these parts of myself. When we hide away our less desirable parts, that quickly leads to feelings like shame and guilt, feelings nobody wants. It is truly reprehensible that for many people their experience of church feels more about trying to elicit feelings of shame and guilt, not lessening them. I am beyond grateful for the very different message I was given.

So if we are all broken, that changes how we see and interact with each other. On good days, when I am able to live out my faith well, I understand that when someone is behaving badly, my job is not to reply with bad behavior of my own, as this will only make things worse. No, my job is to try to understand which crack or imperfection they are speaking from. Once you realize that your own brokenness leads to your worst behaviors then you become aware that is true for others, too.

I know some resist the idea that we are born as anything more than a blank canvas. What good can come from a claim that we are all born with a deficit of brokenness? Maybe that is not the best way to see it. Another perspective I don't think can be argued with is that we are born into an imperfect, cracked, and otherwise broken world. The inevitable outcome of this is that we ourselves will be cracked somewhere along the way.

No matter how we imagine the cause, the universality of brokenness frees us from one very important thing: judgment. We may still compare our scars to others, but we will never encounter anyone who has none. Some of our scars may appear deeper and more obvious, but nobody is free of them. It is not for us to stack our imperfections against others and then declare ourselves the winner or loser.

I have personally found so much freedom in this understanding. I no longer feel so compelled to categorize parts of myself as good or bad because they are all me. Having diabetes and being overweight are part of the total package of being Jeremy. I don't need to be ashamed and treat them like scarlet letters of personal failure because that is both unhelpful and untrue.

As I was listening to the sermons at my newfound church and participating in other adult studies, I was hearing far more than was said. It felt like these messages were being crafted solely for me, though they obviously were not. I was instead tapping into something new in my adult life which my faith tradition calls the Holy Spirit. Call it what you will, it is a source of inspiration and guidance that has helped me better understand the world and my place in it. I discovered I was my own worst critic and what I felt were judgments from others were, in fact, me judging myself. My inner voice had grown overly critical, but now there was a new voice helping me see things about myself I had never seen before.

I learned to think about my choices in life differently as I worked to break free of the harsh cycles of shame and judgment I had put into my life. Which is something I still work on today. Letting go of judgment doesn't mean you no longer worry about consequences. It also doesn't mean you should stop thinking your actions will have consequences or you should stop imposing consequences if someone else's actions warrant them. Far from it. What it does mean is that you cease defining yourself and measuring your value as a person based solely on what you are able or not able to do. You are not a bad person because you ate the whole box of Girl Scout cookies. That is so important it bears repeating. You are not a bad person because you mess up! Stop judging yourself for it. However, you are going to have to deal with the consequence of the cookies, which means a spiked blood sugar.

I have found repeatedly that consequences are so much easier to deal with than judgment. Consequences can most often be repaired; judgment leads to new cracks that often cannot.

I continued my involvement in the same church for the next several years while my wife and I lived in Albuquerque. I formed friendships with others there and learned more about faith, scripture, and God. After about a year a small group started to form among those in the area who worked in youth ministry at the various United Methodist churches in the city. This gave birth to a Friday night house church meeting where we and our spouses would gather. To my great surprise my wife agreed to come with me and it quickly became part of our weekly routine. While we studied various programs and books, it was the people and the relationships that formed between us that were truly transformational. I was becoming a different person and somebody I liked a whole lot better.

I still struggled with my weight and my diabetes, including a period of really poor test results. The difference now was when my A1c was up to 11 percent I had a place to go and talk about it. It was a consequence of some poor choices I was making about what I ate and my activity level and it was serious enough that it demanded attention. I didn't, however, have to deal with it alone. My friends reminded me that my value as a person didn't come from lab results but from somewhere far more important. It came from the love I showed others and the love I received from God.

Being *born again* has been an overused and abused phrase for so long that it has almost no positive meaning left in contemporary culture. So I won't use that. What I will say is that I was different. Over those few years I became a better version of me. I was still me and still broken, but now with scars where once bleeding wounds were. While it may not sound like it, that feels so much better. I liked the person I was becoming, which, for the "always picked last in gym class" fat kid, was a pretty big deal. My faith continues to teach me about myself and others. It has become the lens I look at the world through, and it has given the world a softer hue. I also learned more about the other side of brokenness, which is grace. Grace is the love we show each other even when we don't deserve it. Grace is the love God shows us, no matter how broken or disconnected we feel. Grace from God is not earned but only received, which means the only barrier is our own willingness to receive it. All of these new understandings transformed how I understood life and my place in the world.

I don't know how I could deal with the day-to-day reality of my condition without the concepts of brokenness and grace to guide me. My unfortunately still-common poor blood sugar test would be an oppressive grind on my spirit if I had not learned to show myself the same grace I aim to show others. I don't think I could be vulnerable in the way I need to be to share my story if I didn't understand we were all broken in one way or another. I respect that people will walk different paths when it comes to religion and I will not judge anyone for that. I am, at the same time, so very grateful for the path that I have found.

If you are a person for whom faith or religion isn't part of your life I don't imagine this exempts you from feeling shame and guilt. That was not my experience during the less religious parts of my life.

No matter if you believe you are alive for an intentional reason or by the random happenstance of the universe, the simple truth is that you are indeed alive. That means you are part of the human equation now and you, your life, and all that you don't only impacts you, but a wider than you imagine circle of people around you. The world you were born into is not perfect, far from it. So there is no reason to feel guilty or ashamed when you are not perfect. That is an impossible standard. Instead we all must recognize a fundamental truth: The world gets better and becomes more kind, generous, and tolerant when we do. Are you striving to put more compassion into the world? More kindness? More self-sacrifice? Even if you sometimes fail miserably at it, that's okay, so long as you keep trying.

Diabetes never goes away. Even for those who lose a bunch of weight and get off all the medications it is still there, dormant, waiting to reassert itself. I am honestly jealous of those who manage to get the genie back in the bottle, even if just for a time. I would love to do it myself. But while I continue to face my own struggles, I know I am able to continue the hard work of managing this condition because of the faith that I found.

You are a good person.
You are loved and lovable.
You are like everyone else with cracks and scars.
Those cracks and scars make you, you.

4. Children

Eventually my wife finished up her undergraduate degree and joined me in the working world. Student loans would assure there would be no real change to our household bottom line, but software engineers make a pretty good living so we were fine. As I turned twenty-eight my wife and I felt like we were finally on good footing as a couple after five years of marriage. I now know why divorce is so common in the first five years; it takes about that long to figure out what you are doing. Thankfully we were referred to a wonderful marriage counselor who was able to translate my wife's and my needs to each other.

We both started to feel like the next step was for us to have kids. After all, if things are going well, why not introduce a widely unstable new element to the mix and see what happens? I was sure it would be fun. And, for the most part, it was.

Pregnant wives are different than normal wives and must be treated differently. It became clear to me quickly that my wife was engaged in truly important and difficult work as our son was developing inside of her. My role would be a supporting one as there was no real way for me to help her in what she was doing. For a time this meant automatically driving to the nearby Wendy's for chicken nuggets every time we got in the car. It also meant stopping driving to that same Wendy's when chicken nuggets became emissaries from the devil himself designed to kill any appetite. That is just how things rolled.

As the primary cook in the house, I found it was no small challenge to both assure my wife had what she needed while not overindulging myself in things I knew I shouldn't have. For nine months there were so many overlapping layers of wants, needs, shoulds, and shouldn'ts in our eating, it is a wonder we didn't either starve or blow up like balloons. To be fair, starving was never going to happen, and I did end up putting on some weight along with my wife.

One thing I had to get used to with diabetes was how often I was expected to go to the doctor. Previous to my diagnosis I was not much of a fan of going to the doctor, and it would cause me a great deal of anxiety. So I just didn't go. After my diagnosis I was expected to make appointments two to four times a year, each with a blood draw, whether I wanted to or not. I was just adjusting to this when my wife got pregnant and she started to go even more often than I did.

When you are pregnant your doctor will request many tests including on your blood sugar. Gestational diabetes is a thing that women can get when the already crazy hormones of pregnancy combine to also mess up their blood sugar levels. About one in ten pregnant women develop some form of this condition. It is not any more fun than the other forms of diabetes and is arguably worse because the woman is also pregnant, which is also not fun. Nobody really knows what causes this condition and it often develops later in the pregnancy. If a mother has poorly controlled diabetes before and during the whole pregnancy, that can cause complications for the child.

Gestational diabetes doesn't usually cause serious issues but it can make a person feel like crap and can cause, I am not making this up, "fat baby." Or *macrosomia*, which is far less entertaining to say. Like any form of diabetes, gestational diabetes results in excess sugar in the mother's blood. That sugar gets passed on to the baby and results in him/her getting far more nutrition than he/she needs, which their little bodies store as fat. Oh, how helpful our bodies are. Now this is not medically all that bad, but I have never had to push a whole other person out of my body so I cannot say how big a deal having a bigger-than-expected child is to the mother.

Most women are tested for this condition through a "glucose challenge test," which sounds both awesome and like it should lead to many funny YouTube videos. In reality it is not so exciting. You drink some bad-tasting liquid and sometime later they check your blood sugar level. If your body deals with it well, all is fine. When my wife did her test it came back "borderline." So she took it again with the same result. This would become a bit of a tradition in our home: my wife being *nearly there* on a medical condition I was *all in* on. If she had tried harder, I am sure she could have gotten it over the border. Kidding!

What this did do was make our already complicated food life that much more complicated. Thankfully this latest wrinkle came with an expiration date that would also be, not coincidentally, our son's birthday.

We did come through it and our son was born. Let me just say right here that I love being a dad. Oh, it is hard and my kids make me crazy, but I love it. I really struggle with other guys who talk about being a father like it is a burden or talk down about their kids. I don't get men who wander off and aren't part of their child's life. They are missing out on something amazing!

As much as I like being a dad, from day one it also freaked me out an equal amount. Memories of my own father are dim at best, so I had no clue what the role of a dad was. Was I supposed to be fun or stern? Was "wait 'til your father gets home" going to be a threat or a treat? Both? Neither? I had no clue. That first night in the hospital while holding my son, as my wife rested, I started to apologize to him for having no clue what my job was and not really bothering to think about it much before that moment. This was followed by a classic dad move whereby I put our baby back in the bassinet, told me wife he sort of smelled funny, and promptly left to get us some sandwiches. Thankfully a nurse came into the room shortly thereafter and took care of the obviously dirty diaper.

My son was born a little heavier than expected, so the doctors were concerned. For the two days we were in the hospital they checked his blood sugar level several times to make sure he was just a big baby, not a fat one. You cannot prick the finger of someone this small so instead they poked him on his heel. About half the time he didn't even cry, which I took some pride in. All said and done, it ended up being fine, but I must confess to my own feelings of guilt during the checks. Anyone with a chronic condition worries about passing it down to his or her kids. We all want the best for our children and starting them off with known defective genes feels somehow wrong. This is overstating it, of course, but to a degree it really feels that way. There are so many things I want to pass down to my son, and later my daughter, too, but the finger sticks and daily injections are not one.

My son's arrival both increased my motivation to live and eat better while at the same time increasing my guilt when I failed. I learned a lot about myself after his arrival, including the limits of my patience. Sometimes you just have to put the baby in the playpen and walk away.

My daughter would join the party five years later. By that time we were pros and were home from the hospital in under twenty-four hours. No blood sugar scares with my wife or child this time around, which was a huge relief to me. My wife and I had settled on having two kids because she was an only child and I was a middle child and we both wanted to spare our kids the challenges of being either one of those. Plus, we figured, since we got a boy and a girl we had done our duty and replaced ourselves. This is all parent logic, of course, which doesn't require things to be actually true, they just have to feel true. It is a cousin of politician logic.

As a parent you are responsible for a lot. You will be the primary creator of the environment that shapes the newly arrived clay you've been entrusted with. Kids are born with amazing natural instincts and, looking back, I can see hints of their future personalities even in those first couple months. More is written in our genes than I suspect we even know. Yet for the years your kids are in your home you must make decisions for them that in adulthood they will make for themselves. We had decided long before either child came home to ban real soda from our house. Our children would not grow up with ready access to the bright-red Coke cans I had enjoyed at far too young an age. Fruit juice remains a rare treat, with the constant mantra in our home being, "If you are thirsty, drink water." All of this means our kids actually don't like soda that much. On the rare occasions it is offered to them you can expect half-full cans to greet you on the table in the morning. Genetically speaking, my kids are about an eighth German, so I suppose I shouldn't be surprised.

My kids do crave sugar like ravenous honey badgers, to be fair. We are just doing slightly better than average on the liquid sugar varieties, which is important. Liquid sugar like you find in soda and sweet beverages starts to get absorbed at your tongue, not even waiting for your stomach. It takes almost no work for your body to absorb as it passes almost directly into your bloodstream. This is part of what makes it so very bad for you. The other reason is that it is so very easy to drink way too much. My beloved twelve-ounce can of Coke has about 40 grams of sugar. A similar size serving of fruit juice has in the 35-42-gram range. You would need to eat about ten Jolly Rancher candies to get that same amount. So how fast can you drink a can of soda versus eating ten Jolly Ranchers? Add in the fact that people don't drink just one can of soda a day, and the fact that a twelve-ounce serving is pitifully small in a world of triple Big Gulps, and you start to see the issue. This one difference between my environment growing up and the one my children live in will make a huge difference. Some back of the napkin math (40 grams x 2 a day x 356 days = 29,200 grams = 64.4 lbs.) shows my children will consume over sixty pounds less sugar a year than I did by avoiding the average twenty-four ounces of daily soda I consumed. Sixty pounds!!

Other small changes mean, for instance, my kids have almost never had anything but true whole-grain bread. To them bread is brown, not white. Real whole grain is better because it both has fewer carbohydrates and it takes more work for your body to break it down. It cannot be just absorbed. Your stomach has to work at it for a while, which is a good thing. We've also persisted with bagged school lunches far longer than I ever received.

Starting in seventh grade I got lunch money, and we were allowed to leave the school building at lunchtime. Most days I did one of two things. First, a nearby gas station would sell you two hot dogs or two microwave burritos and a soda for that much. Second, after my town got its first Little Caesars, you could get a slice of pizza, some Crazy Bread, and a soda for the same two dollars. My classmates descended on these two establishments like a pack of crazed hyenas every day. This was my lunch every school day for three years until I could drive to the fast-food places a couple miles away. There it was a wonderland of $2.99 value meals and Taco Tuesday at Taco John's. At the time I thought nothing of it as everyone around me was doing the same thing. The lunch hour saw every purveyor of heavily processed, salt-covered, and sugar-infused "food" overrun by kids at their most important stage of bodily development. It was just what you did.

Even now I have noticed my current town's two Little Caesars locations are parked literally across the street from two of our high schools, and they are places no adult wants to go at lunchtime. So my children will persist with their turkey sandwiches on whole-wheat bread as long as we can convince them to do it. I don't know if it will make any real difference in the end, but we intend to try. We won't repeat the previous mistakes but instead we will endeavor to make new ones.

Parenting in the twenty-first century is very different. My son got his first iPhone at age eight. Not because we really wanted him to have it but because he was starting to be able to stay home by himself for short periods. This was fine except we had ditched our landline phone years ago and we quickly figured out he would have no way to communicate with us or anyone else. Adding a new line to our wireless plan was by far the cheapest option and the iPhone was cheaper than any dumb phone they offered. So there you go. I don't know how anyone who hasn't been trained as a software engineer navigates the parental controls on all the various devices in modern houses, but that has become a big part of my job as a dad.

We were cord cutters before that was even a term when we ditched our cable TV before our son was a year old. We did it to keep our kids away from commercials. Shortly after our son was born I was in the grocery store where I listened to a child throw an epic fit in the cereal aisle. She wanted some puffed carbohydrate and sugarcoated animal-shaped product, of the kind also banned from our house, and was literally quoting the commercial to her poor mom. Like, word for word! This was very concerning to me. At this time we still had cable TV, so I watched the commercials aimed at kids intently and was horrified. Food that barely qualifies as food was being slung at children in incredibly brazen ways. The message was basically, *you will be happy, have fun, and people will like you if you eat this.* For decades beer advertisers have been selling this same message as they abandoned advertising the actual merits of their products and instead show you pictures of happy, attractive people having fun, with the implication being it could be you, too, if you buy their beer. The same is being done to our children. The dangerous part that I knew all too well was that eating these sugar-infused nightmares would, sort of, make you happy. After all, I have a black belt in self-medication via food and know what's possible.

Manufacturers have what they call the "bliss point." This is the point where the maximum amount of salt, sweet, and fat are applied to make food the most enjoyable without going over the top to too salty or too sweet. Seriously, this is a thing! So giant companies engineer food to be maximally attractive and addictive then wrap it up in fun shapes and colors, give it a catchy jingle, then market straight to our children through television commercials that comes over a wire we pay for the privilege to have. So, yeah, before our son was one we cut that cable.

In a world of Netflix, Hulu, and Amazon Prime, being a cord cutter is not much of a big deal so long as you aren't a sports nut, which neither my wife or I am. So there's still plenty of TV watched in our house. What there is not much of is commercials, something that was clearly illustrated when our son was about four years old. We were visiting my wife's parents who at that time had no Netflix but did still have cable TV. About ten minutes after my wife settled our son down with something to watch, he came charging up the steps. "My show stopped!" he insisted, and my wife and I both decided to go to the basement to investigate. What had actually happened was a commercial break. This led to us spending several minutes explaining what commercials were to our son and him being agitated by the whole concept. I took some pride in that.

Today my son would prefer to watch people play video games on YouTube than normal TV. If I were an executive at NBC or another broadcaster, I would be very concerned. YouTube does have commercials because they have to make a buck, but we've never had a screaming fit with either child in the grocery store over cereal, so I am still going to chalk one up in the win column. Disconnecting from the way we have all been conditioned to consume TV might seem extreme to some, and I suppose it is even today. For me it offers something more important: the ability to consume what I want when I want it. I have also noticed I am less likely to watch the truly terrible junk-food-esque TV that many channels seem to be putting out these days. I don't know what TLC stands for now, but the L is certainly not for "Learning" anymore. Turns out there is more than enough high-quality content being distributed today for adequate daily consumption without resorting to *The Real Housewives of the Ozarks* because nothing else is on.

In many ways the relationship I have now with TV is similar to the relationship I wish I could have with food. I don't really want to eat junk food and fall continually victim to the food industry's bliss-point sorcery. Instead I want relatively painless access to quality and nutritious food in reasonable amounts. This is obviously something that is possible to do. Many people actually grew up eating this way so for them it is second nature. To me, it feels like trying to learn to play the violin at age forty. Sure, it is possible, but you'll spend most of the time wishing you had learned it when you were younger. For my kids, my hope and prayer is that it will be at least a little easier for them. I want them to leave our house with more than a handful of pasta-dish recipes and at least a passing familiarity with vegetables. I hope we are getting there but only time will tell.

Kids readjust your priorities in a good way. They force you to be less selfish and make you practice thinking of others. A screaming baby at 2:00 a.m. is a crash course in that. They also help you recognize that no one is an island. We are all connected to other people and we do affect what others think and feel. Studies have shown that even watching someone do a good deed for someone else will make the observer feel better. Though we don't need a study to tell us that; just look at what goes viral on Facebook and Twitter. We are suckers for a feel-good story. This is why learning to love yourself and letting go of things like judgment is so important. It is not just because it is good for you but also because it is good for others!

If you don't have children, that is cool, lots of people don't. But you, yourself, are someone else's child and several somebody else's friend. You are connected to others and when you feel good, that becomes contagious. This is why my faith tradition talks so much about loving your enemies and blessing those who persecute you. Meeting anger with anger just breeds more anger. You damage parts of yourself as you try to damage others. Instead, by returning love for hate you stop the cycle. This goes for your relationship with yourself as well.

It is a cliché but true: my kids have taught me far more than I have taught them. I am a better person because I am their father and I pray often that despite all the mistakes I have made, they see the love that I have for them. Being a parent is a lot of work but never a burden. They may someday develop the same condition I struggle with, but I do what I can to help them avoid it as long as possible. I have the opportunity to help shape a different relationship with food for them than I have.

Though we often keep it to ourselves, having diabetes affects more than just the people with it. It becomes at least a small part of all your relationships. The closer the other person is, say, your child or spouse, the more pronounced it will be. This adds both motivation and anxiety. In the end, though, you can only do so much. Our son has reached an age where he is able to make more of his own decisions about what he eats and how he spends his free time. That needs to happen. But I can't help but worry that I have somehow failed to prepare him as well as I could have. This is just part of the deal when you are a parent. So if you feel the same way, all I can say is, keep doing what you can. In the end that is all any of us really can do.

5. Adult Do-over

Only two weeks after my son was born, Hurricane Katrina hit New Orleans, causing unprecedented damage. While my family was safe, living in the high desert of New Mexico, the company I worked for was about to get handed a whole new challenge. Our company developed software for state and local public health agencies across the country. The main product I worked on was a vaccine registry that tracked individual childhood vaccinations in an effort to increase timely completion of all the required shots. Both the state of Louisiana and the city of Houston were clients and both had unexpected work thrust upon them due to the crisis. When you have lots of people living close together with shared bathroom facilities, like in an evacuation shelter, one thing you worry about a lot is communicable disease. So the shelters in Louisiana and Houston, where many people went, needed to act quickly to make sure things like measles, hepatitis, and rubella did not sweep through the shelters. The only solution to that is vaccination. The question was, who already had their shots and who didn't? Vaccination records are not something people tend to think about before they flee a house filling with water. Thankfully our company's software had exactly the information everybody needed.

About a week after Katrina hit, a call went out for volunteers to go and help do the technical support for the shelters across Louisiana. Despite having a newborn at home, I was very keen to go, and my wife understood. This was a chance to make a real difference, and I desperately wanted to be part of it. I am not sure anyone else campaigned as hard as I did, and I was quickly put on the team. Only a few days after the storm I found myself flying into a place most people were still trying to get out of. Our home base was in Baton Rouge at the headquarters of the televangelist Jimmy Swaggart. For the few hours I could sleep each night it would be on a cot in a small conference room with a portrait of Jimmy hanging over my head. Not kidding.

Each morning, breakfast was prepared by an amazing group of volunteers that kept us well fed. The local Coke distributer had dropped off pallets stacked eight feet high with soda. I would grab a six-pack of Diet Coke each morning on my way to my work area, a small piece of the conference room table inches from my cot. Our first job was to take our registry software, normally deployed on large servers, and shrink it down to fit on a laptop. Dell had delivered a pallet full of new machines and we would go to the makeshift IT center and scoop them up three or four at a time. There was no real time for proper inventory control, so we would write down what we took on Post-it Notes and get on with our work.

Once I arrived, we had thirty-six hours to figure out how to deploy six workstations, a local server, and a printer to each of the vaccine clinics being set up. The goal was to have volunteers print vaccine histories as people checked in so the nurses and doctors would know what to give and what they could skip. In an assessment done later, it was estimated that one million dollars was saved in Houston alone by avoiding vaccinating people who didn't need it.

This was in the early days of common Wi-Fi, so one of the biggest challenges we had was figuring out how to configure the high-end wireless network gear Cisco had sent a crate worth of. There was not much sleeping in those thirty-six hours, which included a run across town to get the data we needed from the main server. No matter how fast your internet connection is, sometimes it is still faster to put it on a disk and drive it.

Once our work was done and we made about a half-dozen copies of the same setup, we were deployed to the various locations. I got to drive a state-owned vehicle across Louisiana full of non-inventoried equipment with no paperwork. For someone who was very used to the slow pace of state government, it was surreal.

The first place I helped set up was the main shelter in Baton Rouge. This is where most people who were at the ill-fated Super Dome site ended up. Where normally there would be basketball and hockey rinks, there were instead rows and rows of cots. Whole families had only a few dozen square feet to share and no real privacy between them and their neighbors. Many of these people were from the Ninth Ward and it was becoming clear they would have nothing to go home to. Their homes, jobs, schools, and neighborhoods were just gone, and many had no idea what to do next.

Some had found a way to upgrade from the standard-issue cot to something more comfortable. There were a smattering of TVs around, usually with large groups of children in front of them. During my day there I noticed some organized activities for the younger people but most of the adults were just sitting. Not really congregating, chatting, or playing cards like I would have expected. Instead they mostly just sat, individually, alone in a very crowded room. Despite the fact there were thousands of people in each shelter, they were surprisingly quiet. There was no huge din of noise like you'd expect from a similar sized group of people attending a sporting event in the same venue. Instead it was just a low murmur as people sat, wondering, I am sure, what the hell they were going to do now.

In the seven days I was there I set up the technology for six shelters of various sizes. Some were in convention centers, some in churches, and some in schools. A couple would be evacuated again shortly after I left as Hurricane Rita swooped in to add insult to injury. Starting with that very first site, after my work was done and the lines were moving, I would wander to where people were staying to talk to folks. If it looked like someone had kids, I made sure to approach them. Kids are who you really worry about getting sick in these situations. I would ask them how they were doing and tell them what we were up to. Despite everyone's best efforts, communication was a problem in the shelters. Things were moving and changing so quickly it was hard to keep track of what was happening when and where. We had people get to the check-in desk after standing in line for sometimes thirty minutes, and only then ask what the line was for. I asked one person why he waited so long if he didn't know why, and he just sort of looked at me and replied, "Because I didn't have anything else to do." So I would talk to parents, tell them why it was important to get their kids vaccinated, and where to go. The times I would see them later in line really made me feel good.

During this week I could not really think about what I was eating and was lucky to remember to take my medication. Sometimes I forgot. I was so caught up in what I was doing that I just didn't want to think about it. I didn't want to be slowed down. So I mostly just ignored it.

Soon my work was done and the local department of health people took over responsibility for setting up the rest of the clinics. I had come there on a one-way ticket, but our company travel agent was able to find me a way home. I was sent south to New Orleans, and would end up taking only the second flight out of the New Orleans airport after it was reopened. The airport had served as a hospital right after the storm and as a place to fly out the most critical patients. When I arrived, there were still cots set up everywhere and it looked more like the backlot for the old show MASH than an airport. Taped to one wall beside one cot was an inflated latex surgical glove that someone had written "Happy 8th Birthday" on. There were five-gallon cans of fresh water everywhere and almost no people. Commercial flights would start with a trickle, with only ten or so scheduled on the departure board for the next twelve hours. Soon I was checked in and through security screening at a speed uncommon in post-9/11 America.

I waited at my gate for over two hours for the scheduled departure. I had no idea what the airport would be like so I arrived early. I stared out the large windows onto the very quiet runways. I noticed armed National Guard troops standing next to my plane and others and I thought about the destruction I had seen on the drive in. Hotels missing walls so that you could see into each room. Destroyed billboards and signs all over. I then realized that I hadn't actually seen the worst of it, far from it. Not knowing what else to do, since I had no smartphone to distract me, I started to pray. "God, what are you going to do with all these people? Who is going to help them?" I wondered. Later I would figure out these were questions best not asked of God unless you are looking to have your life plan messed with, because it was then God spoke to me. Not in a voice, mind you, and there was no burning bush around so far as I could tell, like with Moses, but God was talking more through feelings. As I asked my questions I flashed through all that I had done in the last few days in my mind. I remembered how it felt to talk to strangers about their kids, stay up late working toward an impossible deadline, and the feeling I had at that very moment, sitting in the airport, which was equal parts exhaustion and deep satisfaction. In the language of my faith tradition, I was experiencing a call. I was not sure to do what exactly, but to something. I had no clue what to do with the feelings developing inside of me, so on the flight home I elected to just sleep.

I got home on Friday and was beyond excited to see my wife and son. My in-laws had actually come for a visit while I was gone and we overlapped at the Albuquerque airport for about an hour. So we all gathered in one of the bars, shared a drink, a quick meal, and discussed how absolutely adorable their new grandson was. For the rest of that day and well into the next I slept. When Sunday afternoon arrived I got an email from the owner of the company I worked for. He was impressed by how well our team had done and was giving us all Monday off. I was not going to pass up a free day home with my family. When I did get back to work on Tuesday, my manager called me first thing. She told me again how good the reports were and wanted to let me know I would be getting a bonus in my next check as a reward for all the extra hours. "A bonus?" I thought, "I would have done it for free!"

This whole experience, combined with the addition of my son, sent me on a bit of a journey. I did love the people I worked with and the work that we did. I was not sure you could do better than being both well paid and doing something important like developing tools to help people be healthy. Yet at the same time, I had to confess I began to wonder if my career choice was truly going to be long term. Should I be doing something else? What else was there?

While I was asking these questions, my wife was asking her own. A career in theater, it turns out, is rather hard to have if you also want to have a family. She, too, was wondering if she had made the right choice and if there was something else she should be doing. She actually began her first semester in college premed and there was something about that idea that still lingered. But with a husband and a son, what was possible now? All of these questions swirled around our house for months while we continued to participate in our house church and my wife increasingly realized being a stay-at-home parent was not her long-term ambition. God bless all of you women and men who take that on.

Shortly after New Year's came a turning point conversation. By then my wife had mostly decided that nursing was a route she was interested in and I needed to tell her that I felt a pull toward some sort of career in the church. This was not because I thought the church was all that wonderful, mind you. In fact the church mostly annoyed me at the time and still does. What I saw instead was its potential. As a United Methodist I was learning more about the founder of the Methodist movement, John Wesley, and I really liked his style. There is a quote attributed to him that says, "Do all the good you can. By all the means you can. In all the ways you can. In all the places you can. At all the times you can. To all the people you can. As long as ever you can." What if the church lived into this a little better, I wondered? Could I be a part of helping that happen? If so, what would I do?

I didn't have answers to any of that but I thought I had at least figured out my next step. As an engineer, I had come to appreciate that when you are faced with an important question the first thing you should do is learn all you can about it. I had important questions and I felt called to learn more, which I decided meant going to seminary. After I had finished my undergraduate degree I truly thought school was behind me, but I was wrong. As I shared my discovery with my wife, she was in no way surprised. She had seen this coming long before I did. So within eight months of that conversation I would be enrolled in graduate school and she would be in nursing school. Not only that, but we would be hundreds of miles away, in Ohio, having sold our house and crammed the three of us into a tiny apartment. Our son's first birthday party would be attended by people we had met days prior, and a whole new adventure would be starting.

We had tried being adults, but we were calling a do-over. Time to start again.

Starting over like we were planning to do is never easy. There are all sorts of questions that need answered, like where you will live, how you'll pay for school, how you'll eat, and who will look after your child while both parents are attending class. Some of these questions we had answers for when we arrived in Ohio; others we made up as we went along. Making this sort of switch is hard enough without the extra concerns that having diabetes, or any other chronic medical condition, for that matter, adds to the mix. You see, having diabetes is expensive. There are all the doctor visits, the lab tests, and the monthly prescription drug costs. That alone can be a burden without the extra expense that can occur if any of the longer-term side effects start kicking in. All of this means having good health insurance is a big deal.

We didn't really have any problems in that area while I was pulling in near six figures in income and had a very good group insurance plan through work. At the time I disliked even the $150-a-month premium I was asked to provide, completely unaware of how much my medical care actually cost. In truth, it was the bargain of the century. So as we looked toward not having this type of plan, we began to add up how much me having diabetes was actually costing. I was shocked. I had also assumed that the health insurance plan offered through my new school would be roughly equivalent to what I had before, but I was so very wrong. The difference in the prescription coverage alone would cost us and additional $200 a month at a time when we were planning to live on less than a quarter of our previous income. How was this going to work?

Going without insurance was not an option because the Affordable Care Act had yet to change the rules on preexisting conditions. At the time, any lapse in coverage could mean your new insurer could refuse to cover the cost of any conditions you bring with you. You had to roll from one insurance to another to avoid this. Health insurance, and all the troubles associated with it, is one of the big, underappreciated headaches that comes with a diabetes diagnosis. Many people may have the drive and determination to take their lives in new directions but get caught in a trap when it comes to providing for their health-care needs.

Employer-based plans are great if you have an employer who provides them, but what if you don't? What if you want to start your own business? What insurer is going to give you coverage? People have various feelings about the Affordable Care Act, I know, but at least it tries to give people options. If politicians really want to unleash the creativity and ingenuity of the American people, they'd do well to not overlook the one in ten who have diabetes and need a way to be both entrepreneurial and care for their health needs. The old system we were trying to navigate at the time of this big life transition felt very much like it was designed to keep people dependent on their employers. Where can you go if leaving the safety of the corporate world literally means taking your life in your hands?

Issues with insurance persist now. My wife can tell you any number of stories about what it is like to try to get the medication her patients with diabetes need. Massive amounts of research are being done into new drugs to lower blood sugar, so new products are on the market constantly. Getting these drugs into the hands of the patients who need them is a constant challenge. Many people will leave their provider's office with a prescription that they later find out their insurance company won't pay to fill. Some of these drugs are hundreds of dollars a month, and which insurance company will cover what medication varies.

When you pay for an office visit, you are paying for the time of all the people who help with that visit, not just the provider. The receptionist, nurse, and aides all get paid from that same pot. Today, nurses spend an unreal amount of time doing paperwork for insurance companies or making calls just to get their patients what they need. If you want to know one of the reasons health-care costs are exploding, this is a big one. Nurses and countless other support staff spend hours and hours not helping patients but instead dealing with the bureaucratic mess that is our insurance system. Seriously, the more you know about what is actually going on, the more disgusted you will get.

Within months of our arrival in Ohio we figured out that the plan we had made for health care was unworkable. In the end, it was not me and my issues that did us in; it was our son. After several ear infections his pediatrician informed us the next option was for him to get tubes in his ears. I had this done as a child so it made sense to me. Thankfully Columbus, Ohio has a great children's hospital that could do it in no time. There was just one hitch: it would cost us $4000 out of pocket. The private insurance we bought through the school would only pay about $500 of the expected $4500 cost and the rest was up to us. We had no clue what to do. We vented about the situation to some new friends who were quick to point out that we had overlooked something: Medicaid. Turns out most families living on the seminary campus were on Medicaid. We all made so little money everyone qualified so long as you had kids. In fact, Medicaid would not only cover our son but us as well. It was a health insurance miracle!

We located the right office with the right paperwork and quickly applied. While we were there it was pointed out to us that we would likely qualify for WIC (Women, Infants, and Children food assistance) as well. Government cheese, anyone? Think what you will about these programs, I have no guilt about taking advantage of them. My wife and I had decided to sacrifice a lot to take our lives in a new direction, both because we felt it would be better for us but also because we believed it would help us make the world better. We met and overcame every obstacle put in our way, but when it comes to the poor state of health care in our country, that was a problem far outside our ability to solve. These programs made everything that came after possible, and today when I write the check for our taxes, I am grateful for what we received.

For many people with diabetes, navigating the health-care system can feel like a whole other job. Not only do you have all the diet, exercise, and medication issues to deal with, you also have to become a master at navigating the gauntlet of referrals, pre-approvals, co-pays, and deductibles that come with managing your condition. It is a wonder that more people just don't give up, and I imagine this is why magic cures from outer Mongolia become tempting when they can be summoned with just a couple clicks. For those who work during normal business hours, getting to appointments can be a challenge, and many have to ask for extra time off to do it. Which is something nobody relishes doing.

People with diabetes don't want to be special and different. We want to feel like we can do the same things everyone else can. For the most part that is true, but sometimes it is not. It adds a whole new layer of complication to often already complicated situations. I remember once being two hours into a four-hour drive only to suddenly remember I left my medication at home— medication that cost hundreds of dollars and cannot be easily replaced. I had to turn around. Recently the same thing happened to a colleague and I watched as a group of well-meaning fellow pastors pushed her on why she needed to skip the first part of our Christmas party to run an hour and a half back home. They didn't mean it, but the expression on her face was one I knew well. If it were me, I would be thinking, "Because I am an idiot and thank you all for rubbing it in. Go #@*$ yourselves!" She's a nicer person than me, so I am certain her thoughts were less colorful.

As I write this I can almost be nostalgic for this point in my life and all the adventure that awaited. I can do that because for the most part it worked out well in the end. For many that is not the case. Some choose to be brave and step out on faith only to have their condition beat them back. The extra stress that comes with times like these can mess up your blood sugar. I fear that if I had waited any longer, I might not have been up to the challenge of it all. Thankfully I was still young and foolish enough to leap without really looking.

For a time I was actually considering two different career paths, either pastor or pilot. I took some introductory flying lessons at a local flight school and researched what my employment options would be. Unfortunately, about this same time my doctor was becoming insistent about adding injected insulin to my treatment regimen. Medically it made the most sense of the options I had. It also meant it would be all but impossible to get a job as a pilot because getting a Pilot Medical Certificate is very difficult if you are on insulin. And even if I had one I would be barred from flying outside the United States. Doing the right thing for my diabetes meant closing the door on something I've dreamed of doing for years. The case is similar for commercial truck drivers. If you take insulin to control your diabetes you have to apply for a special exemption that can be a real pain to get.

If you are struggling with our broken medical system, I feel for you. Know your doctors and nurses understand and they are frustrated, too. If you are being held back from doing what you want by the cost of your medications, I get where you are coming from. If your condition is limiting you from following your dreams, trust me, I know that sucks. These are real and hard issues.

All I can say is, don't give up. The world needs each person in it and that includes you. We don't often see the solutions to our problems until they are right in front of us, which is either exciting or supremely annoying depending on your perspective at the moment. Either way, remember that you are more than your condition and you make a difference to others every day, even if you don't see it.

6. The Subcontinent

Our adventure in Ohio was off and running as we settled into a four-year marathon of classes, child raising, and unfamiliarly low levels of discretionary income. My wife thrived in her program while I adjusted to a very unfamiliar routine of reading many books and writing lots of papers. In college I had written exactly one paper for one class and I got a D. I felt woefully unprepared for the work I was being currently asked to do. Most classes required several writing assignments and sometimes up to half a dozen books to read. My first semester I was just barely keeping my head above water. I was so very thankful that my wife had developed a far better grasp of written English than I had. She understood where to put commas and the difference between where/were and their/there/they're. Everything I wrote had to be done at least a day early so she could review it and make sure my appalling grammar was not overshadowing the thoughts I was trying to convey. We were quite a team.

Between the move, the stress of school, and all the other things we had going, my weight started to go up after being stable for years. I didn't feel like I was eating all that badly, and in fact our new financial condition meant that the several meals a week we formerly were eating at restaurants were now eaten at home. This had to have a positive impact on my diet, I reckoned. Despite that, I was gaining weight. So I did the only logical thing I could: I stopped getting on the scale. That would be reserved for my biannual doctor's visits, figuring I was going to get a lecture either way, so what was the big deal.

I was still consulting a little on the side for my old company because the money was just too good. The challenge was keeping my income under the limit for Medicaid because crossing that boundary would bring far more pain than benefit. Add to that I had been recruited into an internship at a local church, basically to be very cheap technical support. Between the jobs and class I was busy, and my wife's schedule was not much better. We lived on the campus of my school and she had to commute to her's. Her clinical hours were done all over the area including an interesting maternity rotation at the local county jail. Our son spent more time than we would have liked at a nearby day-care center. It was mostly populated by children of upper-middle-class folks, and the monthly fee was more than our rent. We wanted him to have the best, though, because of the three of us, he had no choice in our little adventure.

As big as an adventure as this was becoming, there was a piece of fine print I hadn't thought much about when we arrived at the seminary. The school I was attending required every student in my program to participate in a cross-cultural experience. These were trips lead by faculty that went various places. Some went to closer by places, like visiting Native American reservations in the West. Having spent most of my life near several reservations in Montana and New Mexico, that was not very interesting to me. Some trips went to farther-flung places, and I elected one of those: India. Before the opportunity for the trip came up, I never thought much about India. I knew jobs from my previous career were being shipped there as more and more tech companies were setting up outposts in places like Bangalore, but that was about all I knew. The pre-immersion classes didn't help much as they purposely kept us in the dark about what we could expect. They wanted us to experience it clean and not through predetermined lenses. This was all fine by me. It meant less reading.

The trip lasted a little less than three weeks and we visited none of the touristy places from TV. We didn't see the Taj Mahal or the Himalayas. We stuck to southern, more rural India where few western tourists go. It would not be an understatement to say the trip changed my life. It could be a book by itself easily. It was worth every nickel and minute spent on it and then some.

For obvious reasons journeys like this have added layers when you know you'll have health conditions to manage along the way. After I committed to the trip but before we went, I was put on a new medication. This medicine was injected, which meant giving myself twice-daily shots. It also had to be kept below a certain temperature, which added complications. Finally, and most importantly, it had introduced something new into my life: low blood sugars.

I have said already high blood sugar levels can make you feel a little icky or achy, but are generally not a big deal in the moment you are having them. Low blood sugars are a whole other thing. Remember, your body runs on sugar; it needs it to function. When your sugar is low, your body notices and reacts. It was not uncommon at this time for me to be woken up in the middle of the night feeling very strange. The only way I can describe it is feeling very hungry and tipsy at the same time. Your muscles don't want to work and you brain is running at half speed. All parts of your body, including your brain, are competing for the limited amount of fuel running through your system. On one occasion I could not even get out of bed and had to wake up my wife to help me.

The treatment for low blood sugar is straightforward: eat or drink something. This was the rare time I was glad to have fruit juice in the house. Your body is an amazing machine and can recover quickly if you have the right things on hand. The big challenge is not overdoing it and sending your level into the stratosphere. That is no good either. Most times this happened to me at night, which is honestly preferable to the couple of times it happened in class or the one time it happened while driving. So India would offer an interesting challenge.

I am pretty sure that, at the time, stress and diet meant my blood sugar was all over the place. My A1c test was up, thus the new medication, and it had the desired effect of bringing my average down. However, this particular medication also made my rare low times even lower, causing the new issues. I was right to be worried about what this would mean for me on the trip. If this was happening while I was home and had ready access to foods I knew I liked, what would it mean when that was gone and I was presented mostly with foods I was pretty sure I would not care for? As adventurous as I can be when it comes to travel, that sense of daring does not often extend to food. At this point in my life I was a pretty narrow eater and I didn't expect to encounter much from my preferred list while we were there.

My wife was concerned, too, and together we crafted a strategy. Some of the very limited space in my luggage would be given over to protein bars. Now, most of these bars would be better termed carbohydrate bars, given how much sugar they contain. Most of the time they should be avoided by anyone with diabetes, but this was the rare exception. We figured as I ate through my supply of bars, that would create space for souvenirs. We applied similar logic to the stash of toilet tissue and Kleenex I would also be bringing along that were important for other reasons. Both the bars and the tissue turned out to be lifesavers.

A trip like this demands you go with the flow. We had been given a broad overview of the trip but the actual day-to-day schedule would be spooned out over the days and weeks. Part of the reason for this was that sometimes the leaders honestly didn't know when things would happen. India is a crowded, moving, and dynamic country, even in the more rural southern part. Sometimes plans just had to change and it was easier to do that if the whole group was not holding tight on to detailed itineraries. This added an element of surprise and uncertainty I personally enjoyed. A few other people felt like I did and we would find ways to use any unexpected holes that developed in our schedule. This included taking an unchaperoned ride in a pair of auto-rickshaws out of the safety of the Church of South India Seminary we were staying at, into town, to the train station, where we were told we could expect to find coffee. It was great fun. When we returned a couple hours later several of our group were right where we left them, playing cards. To each their own.

This trip happened just before iPhones and Facebook changed the way we interact. Communicating home meant either using something akin to a pay phone or suffering through very unreliable dial-up internet access to send an email. I talked with my wife as often as I could, but there was no escaping that you were truly *away*. I had to deal with my reality and had no choice but to let the homesickness subside and give in to the experience. This kind of true immersion may not even be possible now, as wireless service is nearly universal; if so I am not sure that is a good thing.

Consistent blood sugar monitoring and very gracious hosts meant the worst possible scenarios for my diabetes didn't come to pass. After a couple days I ditched the injected medication, discovering there was no practical way to keep it at the right temperature. My blood sugar level would be higher than it should be, but that was just part of the cost of the trip. I hoped the couple of weeks would be short enough to cause no harm in the long run. I decided not to mention this to my wife in my calls home. While one of our group would end up in the hospital, it would not be me. Instead, between the bars I brought with me and a slowly adapting palette, I avoided all but one bad low blood sugar episode, and even that was easily dealt with. That, however, didn't mean issues didn't arise in different places.

One day we were crowded into a bus and sent off to see… something. I honestly don't remember what. I do remember that as I was departing the bus, our faculty leader, Tim, asked me how I was feeling. He genuinely was trying to be helpful as he gave me a reminder that I need to care for myself and asking if I needed something to eat. He was one of the few who knew I had diabetes and perhaps the expression on my face tipped him off that something was amiss. The truth was I was feeling a little off and I had also grown tired of my limited protein bar flavor options. I had one with me but I was not keen to eat it. What Tim had meant as concern I took all wrong.

Again, people with diabetes don't want to be special or treated differently. We don't want to be singled out and would prefer to suffer in silence, *thank you very much.* Add to the mix that no overweight person wants to ever be asked, *do you need to eat?* Aren't I carrying enough extra with me? I mean, really, should my body even need food for the next several years given what I already weigh? When you are already tired and a bit worn down, your mind just jumps to crazy places like this. So I snapped back with a quick, biting comment and stormed off. Thankfully Tim is a gracious person so no real harm was done. Yet I still remember the experience and I am not proud of it. When things like this happen, your mind, for no useful reason, stores them away in a place easily retrieved. So they are always there to remind you that you're not perfect.

A few days later there would be a similar incident over some chips. After making a comment to nobody in particular about my desire for a snack, our local host decided to try to meet the request at our next stop. When we pulled over he turned around, looked at me, and asked me if I would like him to get me some chips. At this point I already had a reputation among the group for not being the most adventurous eater, and that combined with all my normal fat-person shame. Like hell he was going to go to any special trouble to find me an obviously unhealthy food option just because I was too picky to eat what I was served. So I quickly retracted my request and stared at the floor. Shortly afterward, someone else popped up and cheerfully said, "Chips sound good, I will have some." Well, I thought, if others were going to do it then that is different. So I started to add my order to the mix.

Tim would tell me later that he had known our local host for years. He was a professor of theology in India and in the United States where Tim had studied. He had been with him on these types of trips before and counted him a good friend. Never, Tim explained, had he ever seen our host as mad as he was in that moment. Changing my mind and making this very simple thing overly complicated was not only annoying but it also crossed local cultural lines. In India, you don't really tell people flat-out no. It is impolite. When I said no and then went back on it that was a big deal. You just don't do that. Our host actually did a good job muting his anger in the moment, but it was clear I had crossed a line. I went back to staring at the floor.

Giving in to weakness never feels good. Not after it is over and not in the moment. That is what this felt like. Like a known alcoholic casually suggesting, *why don't we all go get some drinks?* Even if nobody else saw it that way, that is the way it felt in my head. Should someone choose to register displeasure with the request or offer a subtle eye roll at the fat guy with diabetes giving in to a carb craving, all the worse. The shame spiral that would likely follow would be epic. So, yeah, I just kept staring at the floor.

These were two small moments in an otherwise brilliant trip. There were countless highs to more than balance out the lows, and then some. As our time drew to a close I knew it had been worth it. Our last stop was Chennai, and from there we would fly home. We took a train to get there and it was a true experience for at least one of us. At this point I knew the people in our group far better than I did when we started out. One friend I had made was Allen, and he had the distinction of being the only one of us destined to go on to get a PhD. He is brilliant. He was always up for a theological debate and the trip offered no shortage of opportunities. Allen and I could be often found conversing about the deeper parts of Christian thinking or playing chess on a small board purchased near the train station where we searched for coffee. Unfortunately for Allen, he also had the distinction of being the only one of our group to get really sick. Like, in-the-hospital sick.

When we arrived in Chennai most of the group went to the YWCA where we would be staying, while Allen, Tim, and I headed to the hospital. Allen and I would stay the night, mercifully in a private room, and rejoin the group the next day. The doctors and nurses were quick to treat Allen's obvious stomach ailment and he was feeling better quickly. Even a power outage in our room didn't deter the nurses from getting their blood draw. This is apparently not uncommon. The visit ended up costing only about $100 and Allen earned some extra bed rest back at the hostel we were staying at. The next day our group went ahead on that day's trip and I found myself with not much to do as Allen slept.

At this point I was ready to be home and was more than happy to have some time to myself. I wandered out of the hostel and down the main road. There was a shopping center, tons of traffic, and people everywhere. This city was hopping. Eventually it got to be after lunch and I had no idea what I should do. I assumed the YWCA would feed us but it was a long walk back. Instead I had another idea. A block away I spotted a large congregation of auto-rickshaw drivers and made my way to them. A few came over to me as I approached. "I want some American food," I said to them. They looked at me quizzically so I repeated it. Most folks in India do speak English, so that was not the problem, it was just a bit of an unorthodox request. A few of them discussed among themselves, not in English, and finally one pointed to his vehicle and said, "Okay. Get in." So I did.

A couple of things to understand at this point. First, I had forgotten to ask the price upfront, which we were told to always do. So I was going to get gouged. Second, and more importantly, if you ever wondered what people mean when they talk about *white male privilege*, this is it. Here I was, wandering the streets of a country I still didn't understand, asking locals to solve my problem for me, and assuming I would be safe and well treated while they did. Any woman on our trip could not have done what I did with such confidence. She would have had to worry about a whole universe of possibilities I didn't have to. This is similar to our regular practice of teaching college girls how not to get raped instead of teaching our boys not to rape girls. It is just assumed that women inhabit a world where being raped is a possibility while men don't. That is quite a privilege we men have. This whole conversation deserves more time than I can give it, but I could not let this moment go by without bringing it up.

The driver took me on a couple-mile ride and then charged me about four times what it should have cost. He pointed toward a set of double doors leading to a set of stairs into the basement. After traversing a small hallway, the place I had been delivered to came into focus. It was a restaurant. It had a hostess stand, normal-looking tables and chairs, and the decorations made it look like a knockoff Applebee's. Sparky's had been opened by a Hawaiian expat to serve the American businessmen who were flooding into India. I was seated at a table with inlaid memorabilia from Montana, the state I spent most of my childhood in. Sitting a couple tables down were two software engineers from Oracle who knew some of the people from the first company I had worked for out of college. The menu featured burgers, fries, Coke products, and a French dip, which I ended up ordering. I knew in that moment God was real and wanted me to be happy.

I didn't care that I was missing whatever it was the rest of the group was seeing. I am sure it was interesting but I was exactly where I wanted to be. I took over an hour to eat my lunch. I relished every bite and left feeling like I had the energy to get through the last couple days. The same driver was waiting for me when I got out and he was more than happy to take me back to where we were staying. He charged me quadruple again but I didn't care. When I got back to our room Allen was asleep so I joined him. A good meal and a nap. I was in heaven.

Reunited with the rest of the group that evening, I shared with them my adventure. At this point most pretense had been dropped and even those who were attempting to stay as native as possible in their eating joined me there for lunch the next day. My biggest regret of the trip was not buying a souvenir hat from Sparky's like others in the group had. A Google search shows it is closed now and a search for *American Food* turns up more places like KFC and Pizza Hut than I ever saw years ago. That makes me kind of sad.

Comfort food is not just advertising jargon—it is a real thing. We all have tastes and smells that bring us to somewhere else in an instant. They come from the same part of the brain that controls memory, which makes sense if you think about. In the hunter-gatherer days of our species it would be very important to remember where the food was found. Even years later, ancient humans could reenter a valley and remember, *the good berries were over there!* That is an important skill to have.

Comfort food will vary from culture to culture and family to family. We like what we grew up eating and when we are older we remember the happy times when we eat it. This includes those moments when the food itself is the happy thing we remember. I can still take down a whole brick of graham crackers given the opportunity and enjoy every minute of it. I suppose people raised on kale and quinoa can have good feelings associated with foods like that. For most of us it is more likely pancakes, fried chicken, or mom's spaghetti. Having diabetes reorients your relationship with food in such a way that even cherished childhood memories are called into question. My standard dinner request for my birthday or other special occasion growing up was lasagna. It is one of the few inherited recipes I have that I resisted tampering with. It is just too important that it be made just so. But all those layers of white pasta have become a no-no for me. I know full well what will happen with even a single piece. So it is a rarity in my house now. Such a rarity, in fact, that my children don't care for it much and turn their noises up at the sliced hardboiled egg on top (you're just gonna have to trust me on that part.) On a rational level, I know that is not a bad thing. On an emotional level, it hurts.

I have my favorite pizza place, barbeque place, and sandwich joint. We all do. A big challenge for anyone with diabetes is to figure out where the line between occasional indulgence and potentially dangerous overindulgence is. The morning after Christmas day my blood sugar was pretty bad. That is understandable. It needs to be not so bad on the twenty-seventh or twenty-eighth of December, however. The Super Bowl calls for pizza and nachos while every Monday night football game does not. This is all the more difficult as the food you love can be increasingly summoned via a phone call, web click, app download, or even text. The menus hanging on our fridge remind us of what we could be eating instead of the kale and quinoa. We navigate all of this while we confess sometimes we just need the French dip because the preceding days have been so difficult, and we need the comfort of the familiar.

If you are in a season of life where you are giving in more than you should to the need for comfort, know this: you are forgiven. It happens to us all. It is not always as obvious as a trip to the other side of the world. Sometimes it is just many little things adding up to something that feels big. Whatever the reason, I get it. We all have these times. You cannot stay there forever, mind you! The shorter the better, in fact. But give yourself a break when you pull off to the rest area of comfort food. It will do you no good to beat yourself up for it. Instead, find your way back out onto the correct road as soon as you can.

7. The Liquid Lunch

The last year of our adventure in Ohio was going well. We had planned for two children and we were keen on them being somewhat close together in age. Going back to school had gotten in the way of those plans, so we developed a new plan where my wife would graduate pregnant if possible, but not so pregnant it got in the way of her finishing school. Typically planning like this is foolhardy, but for us it actually worked out. In June, when she got her diploma and pin (it's a nursing thing) she would be a few months into her pregnancy. It also became clear in that last year that she would not stop where she was and wanted to continue on to get her master's in nursing and become a nurse practitioner. This would also turn out to be easier than expected when she was accepted into a program back in Montana where we would be heading next.

Nurse practitioners (NPs) are often lumped in with physician's assistants (PAs) and called *mid-level providers*. Depending on what state they live in, it will vary how much they are allowed to do. In some, mostly southern, states they cannot do much more than what a normal nurse can do. Out west, especially in the northwest, NPs are often fully independent providers who can treat, write prescriptions, and do minor clinical procedures like stitching and lancing. Oh, the stories she can tell about lancing things. PAs are a little different because while an NP will have his or her own license, a PA always works under the license and authority of a physician. Practically, though, they are often treated similarly in large clinics and hospitals.

Multiple studies have shown that NPs are as effective or more effective than physicians in the areas they work in. NPs, and PAs, too, have a narrower scope of things they can do, but in those scopes they have proven again and again to be as good for patients as full medical doctors. NPs and PAs are a godsend to rural areas that could never attract a physician. There is a growing shortage of general practice doctors; all the big doctor money is in specialties, you see, and NPs and PAs are filling that gap. About once a year I see my doctor; the rest of the time I see the NP he works with. In the parts of the US where NPs are not given the same authority to practice as they are out west, you have to wonder why. Or at least you do until you remember that medicine is full of politics like everything else.

My wife had her next stage figured out and I also knew where I would be heading. In January I got the call that the bishop intended to appoint me to serve a small church in Montana's largest city. We were both excited. This would be going home for us in many ways, but it would also be a brand-new adventure. The only thing that hung over me was the realization that the last three years had taken a toll on my body. The crazy schedule, the constant deadline of papers, and the fact that I had decided to become a student pastor for two very small congregations was not leaving a lot of time for me or managing my diabetes. Some new drugs added along the way kept my blood sugar levels at bay but I found myself pushing 300 pounds, heavier than I had ever been. I had to move from XXL to XXXL in most things and I tried very hard not to think about it. If I did, I would likely cry.

Fed up with where I was, I resolved to talk over options with my doctor at my next visit. I told him I was tired of how I felt and looked and wanted to know what I could do. He commented that I seemed far more determined than he had ever seen me. We talked a little about weight-loss surgery but the cost alone made it unworkable. He then suggested a clinic that did a meal-replacement program. I was intrigued. These types of programs are basically the closest you can get to quitting eating cold turkey. All decisions about what you eat are removed, and you are put on a very restrictive diet composed entirely of meal-replacement drinks. Because it is so drastic, I had to visit the clinic weekly and my medication was being constantly adjusted, meaning reduced. I liked that. My personality can be all or nothing, so the fact that I no longer had to think about what I was eating was something I took to quickly.

I still prepared most meals for my family; I just didn't eat them, which was only weird at first. I also found that the chocolate drink powder mixed in Diet Coke was actually quite good. This whole process was not cheap because the clinic was out of network for my insurance. But we made it work and the weight started to come off. After a couple of months, I was asked by a nurse at the clinic what my goal was and I replied, "I want to weigh what it says on my driver's license." She laughed. I got my license at fifteen so it said I weighed 225, which was likely a lie even at that time. Strangely every time I renewed it or moved states they just copied the number over without question. So there it sat, in my wallet, taunting me.

I spent about six months on the program, visiting the office weekly, and leaving with that week's supply of pouches. I didn't really tell anyone I was doing it and simply avoided meeting people for meals. I learned to drink my coffee black and since most people were used to seeing me with a Diet Coke in my hand anyway that was no big deal. At one point I did take a trip with some fellow students to Nebraska to present a paper we had written. There was no hiding it from them, but they were gracious. I did go off-diet for one meal while we were there and, boy, did it taste good. What I remember most from that trip was the flight there. I had never fit so well in an airline seat. Why hadn't I done this before!?

For many people, a meal replacement program works like it did for me. While you are doing it, you simply forget that all the rest of the food options exist. Life gets much simpler, and you just go with the flow. Even Oprah once did the same program I was doing when she famously attempted to get into her skinny jeans. Like me, she did lose the weight. Even I have seen the clip on YouTube of her coming out wearing her goal pants.

The practice my wife works for now is a combination of endocrinology and medical weight loss. She works with patients who are managing their diabetes and with those preparing for the various forms of weight-loss surgery or other programs her department offers. Despite the fact that many hospitals and clinics now offer a version of the meal-replacement program I was on, her office doesn't. They don't do it for the same reason I would have trouble recommending it to others. While you're on the program it is likely going to be fine, but eventually you will need to go off, and that is where the trouble starts. All the temptations you were ignoring for those weeks or months are still there. The country didn't fall out of love with high-fructose corn syrup even though you were not partaking. And, for me anyway, the animal part of my brain I had always been fighting about food with was still there, just hibernating. As I started to ease back into eating real food, I realized I was not wading into the shallow end but jumping off the high dive. I was ill-prepared to swim. Those with stronger wills than I could likely navigate it better. I didn't do well.

It was not a total failure in the months that followed, but it was not a success either. I had read the literature I was given about eating better, but I didn't have a way to practice it when my food was all coming in powder form. I had arrogantly stated over and over while I was on the program that I was not going through all that trouble just to gain the weight back later. I was wrong. Mind you, I didn't gain it all back, but I did some. After we moved to Montana and I found a new doctor, some of the medications had to come back. I hated that more than I did the weight. It eventually settled at about 270, which was less than when I started but far more than my low of 220. I take some comfort in the fact that with all the resources at her disposal, even Oprah could not keep the weight off long term and would struggle like the rest of us.

Every day I see something about the diet of the moment. Someone is constantly claiming that they have discovered the secret of losing weight while still getting to eat like we have grown accustomed to. I remember the Atkins Diet, the South Beach

Diet, and all the rest. For some they worked, and if you encounter one of those people they won't let you go without telling you about it. I get the impulse—they are trying to help. They found something that worked for them and they want to share it. But what if it doesn't work for you? Does that mean you are a failure? Part of the issue with the program I had tried was that the support ended just as I needed it most. One of the reasons Alcoholics Anonymous works is that you don't do it alone. You are part of a community that supports you. Not even my friends could help because I hadn't told them what I was doing.

So despite my good intentions and the work I had done, pounds slowly started to creep back on. I was not suddenly in love with vegetables and after denying myself for so long it was easier than ever to justify indulging in what I shouldn't. The other thing I failed to do well when I was on the program was up my activity level in the way I needed to. This all meant that the weight and drugs were bound to come back.

Diabetes drugs work in various ways in your body and some can actually *cause* weight gain, which is counterproductive long term. Metformin, which can go by several brand names, is typically the first drug someone gets prescribed when they are diagnosed with type 2 diabetes (it doesn't do anything for people with type 1). It has been available since the 1950s and is proven both safe and effective. Metformin doesn't work on your pancreas as you might expect; it actually works on your liver. One of your liver's many jobs is to help regulate how much sugar is in your blood. It will release sugar when it senses you are getting too low, such as between meals, and it is supposed to stop after you have eaten something and your digestive system kicks into gear and starts putting sugar into your blood. For people with diabetes, the signals to your liver can get messed up. It will still produce even after sugar is coming into your blood through other means. This can lead to high blood sugar and, thus, diabetes. Metformin curtails your liver from releasing too much sugar and brings down your overall blood sugar level. For folks with typical type 2 diabetes, Metformin is something they will likely take forever. Thankfully it doesn't cause low blood sugars, and it doesn't cause weight gain. If you do well with your diet and exercise, it could be the only drug you need to take. If that is the case for you then I am extremely jealous.

As the rates of diabetes have increased, so have the number of more complicated cases. Metformin is now often not enough for people, and several different types of drugs are on the market now. One type of drug common today is called *Sulfonylureas*. It goes by several brand names, but does the same thing: stimulate your pancreas to produce more insulin. More insulin in your blood means more sugar gets absorbed by your cells, and your blood sugar level goes down. So you can see the appeal. However, the potential issues should also be apparent. Cells absorbing more sugar means more sugar getting absorbed everywhere, including your fat cells. Also, insulin production now is being artificially influenced and your body's natural systems are not fully in charge. So these types of drugs can lead to both weight gain and low blood sugars. When I was prescribed one of these drugs, I was asked about low blood sugars but the weight gain aspect was never explained. Given that most general practice providers are allotted only fifteen minutes per patient, it's no wonder a lot of useful education doesn't happen. The other issue with this type of drug is, how effective is it to whip an already tired horse? If your pancreas is not working 100 percent correctly, why put extra stress on it?

Now you may be asking, why are these drugs even out there? Well, simple: because sometimes they are what works. The exact set of circumstances that leads to a person having type 2 diabetes varies. Some may be more insulin resistant overall. Some might have pancreas issues. Some might have more of a liver problem. Depending on what combination of a lot of factors causes your diagnosis, different drugs may be appropriate. Treating diabetes is always a trade-off. One drug might cause low blood sugars, but how does that compare to the possibility of diminished eyesight, which can come from prolonged high blood sugar? These are the trade-offs people with diabetes are constantly asked to make. This is why it is critical to see your medical provider often and be clear with them about your goals. I hit a point where being 270 pounds was no longer acceptable to me and I was willing to take the risk of higher sugar levels for a time while I worked on my diet and exercise. So I came off one drug and went on another.

The painful truth is that all drugs have risks. What you have to decide is, when is the risk worth it? The challenge is that even with wildly uncontrolled blood sugar you can feel fine. So why risk taking anything? Well, while it is true that you may not be noticing any bad side effects day to day from your diabetes there will come a day when you do, and it will be bad. Like, blindness, cutting off your foot, or dropping dead of a heart attack bad. Having diabetes can feel all or nothing. Either no big deal or literally life and death, with very little in between. I, like most people, don't like contemplating the worst-case scenarios, so I don't. Instead I go to the doctor, take my pills, try to be good about what I eat, and pray like crazy to avoid the worst my condition can do to me.

Today, there are all sorts of new types of drugs on the market. With over 8 percent of the world population having some form of diabetes, it is a good-sized market. Billions of dollars are spent each year on research. We now have drugs that will cause your kidneys to extract more sugar from your bloodstream and thus bring down your levels. This is good, because it won't cause low blood sugar or weight gain, but not so good that it gives your kidneys more work to do. Other drugs slow the speed at which food leaves your stomach because leaving too quickly can elevate your blood sugar. This has a side benefit of making you feel fuller longer and can even allow for easier weight loss. These drugs are also injected—no fun—and often expensive. Everything has a trade-off, with some being certainly better than others.

All of this is why you need to be as informed as you can as a patient. I was guilty for a long time of just taking whatever my doctor handed out, not asking many questions, and generally being uninvolved in the whole process. The problem with this is, I was the one taking the drugs, not my doctor. Most of the time I didn't even know what the drugs did, so when unplanned side effects did come up I had no clue which of the white, similarly shaped pills I was taking was responsible. This is not the right way to do things. I realize nobody is looking for more things to do. Reading the literature that comes with your drugs is not exactly compelling. Yet most of what you need to know is available to you easily, through your pharmacist. Pharmacists are unsung heroes in the medical world and know a lot of things you need to know. Anytime I get prescribed something new I always ask the pharmacist about it.

It is not uncommon for my wife to come home frustrated at her patients. She complains that they will sit in her office, nod along as she talks, then leave and do nothing she asked them to do. I don't often think about it from the provider's perspective because I am always the one sitting on the exam table. For me it feels like an interrogation that I have paid for the privilege to have. Things move so quickly in a modern clinic, there is little time for chitchat and it's straight to business. Well, when that business is evaluating how well you are managing an oftentimes unmanageable-feeling situation, it is hard for it to be a warm and fuzzy experience.

The other thing that drives my wife a little crazy is all the excuse making. She went on a bit of a rant at the dinner table once about people whom she suspects think they will somehow get a free pass if they can make excuses for all the hard things they are being asked to do. "It's as if they believe I have a secret, easy answer I am hiding from them!" she said in exacerbation. I had to contain my laugh because all I could think was, *yeah, we do kinda think that*. Some of us are hoping there will be a cure soon that will just make all this go away. Some of us are ignoring our condition on the hope that new therapies will come soon enough before any real damage is done. Some of us think we are especially burdened by life and deserve special treatment. We all think these things. So, yeah, break out the good stuff from Canada and let's get on with this.

Unfortunately, as we all know, while drugs might be cheaper in Canada, they have the same stuff we do. I want to believe in magical solutions that will manage my blood sugar and let me frequent HomeTown Buffet guilt free, but it is not going to happen. We are stuck with the trade-offs for the foreseeable future. I will keep praying for the day the magic pill arrives, and I will personally start the bonfire of every copy of this book when it does, but until then betting your long-term health on some future magic cure is about as sensible as betting your whole retirement fund on black at the high-limit roulette table in Vegas. Sure, you could do it, but I cannot recommend it.

You are right; going for diabetes checkups is no fun. Keeping track of your medication, remembering to take it, and learning about what in the hell it is actually doing to your body takes time you'd rather spend on anything else. God only knows how good we would all be at underwater basket weaving if we could have that as a hobby instead. But you have to keep doing it. Like saving for retirement or paying off credit cards, the long-term benefits are just too great. I heard once on the radio that people with children were not statistically happier than people without children. However, people with grandchildren were greatly statistically happier than those without them. My kids are already amazing, and I plan to be around to see how amazing their kids are and reap the happiness benefits of all our hard parenting work. The truth is, I am not just doing this for myself; I am doing it for them. I am doing it for my wife. I am doing it because there is so much out there that is out of my control, so I am going to do what I can with the parts I can control. And that is all any of us can do.

8. Infernal Contraption & The Blue Pill

The first few years we were in Montana are a bit of a blur. In there somewhere our daughter was born, on a Sunday like a good pastor's kid. Somehow our son got old enough to start school, and my wife finally finished hers. First she took the job she could get. Then about a year later, she got the job she wanted. She actually did her master's thesis on diabetes, so when the position she ultimately got came open she was pretty excited. I was thrilled by her steady paycheck because while pastors do okay, they don't make near what software engineers do. We could finally make progress on the chronic condition we both now shared: student loans.

While I worked to be the best pastor I could to the church I had been appointed to, I found a new doctor and continued the never-ending process of managing my condition. Medications came and went, and I endeavored to walk more while also discovering that asparagus, something I have avoided my whole life, really was not all that bad. I guess all those people eating it weren't crazy. As I continued to visit my doctor, a new form started to show up and new questions kept being asked, all about how I slept. In the beginning I was not sure what to make of all this newfound interest in my sleeping. As far as I knew, I slept fine. I certainly appreciate a good nap now and then, especially on Sunday afternoons, but that is really all preachers. Even my dentist got into the act, subjecting me to the same sleep questionnaire I had received from my doctor. Look, I am a busy guy, if I look tired, that is why.

Or was it?

What each of them was after was to screen me for something called sleep apnea. Sleep apnea happens when your breathing interrupts your sleeping, sometimes hundreds of times a night. It happens for a couple of reasons: either your throat muscles fail to keep your airway open so it gets blocked, or your brain fails to signal your lungs to breathe as often as it should. Either way, your body is starved for oxygen for a short time, parts of your brain wake up, and your heart goes into panic mode as it tries to move more blood with less oxygen in it. All of this happens while you're still asleep, so you don't notice it. As you might expect, this is bad for you. Good stress on your heart like from a solid twenty minutes on the treadmill is one thing. This is bad stress on your heart, like someone jumping out and scaring you several times a night. But again, you're asleep, so you don't notice.

Sleep apnea is common for both people with diabetes and those who are overweight. Two strikes against me right there. When my doctor first brought up his concern I was not excited. First, I felt fine. Second, I didn't like the possibility of having another serious condition that I could not really see or feel. Third, the only effective treatment was a Darth Vader sounding mask I would have to use every night to keep my airway open. No thanks on all counts, Doc, sorry.

I ignored my doctor on this for a year, until my wife came with me to an appointment and he drafted her into the effort. I finally relented and took a referral for a sleep study. This is a wonderful process where you get to spend the night at the hospital, hooked up to a bunch of sensors while the machines and a camera watch to see if you stop breathing. If you do, and do it a lot, they'll wake you up in the middle of the night and apply the Darth Vader mask to see it if helps. Oh, and depending on insurance it can be expensive. So, you know, that is all lots of fun.

In our area, the sleep center was really behind so my appointment was not for a couple months. Now, I am not proud of this next part, but it is true. When the reminder call came a week prior to the study I realized my wife had forgotten about it so I canceled. It didn't come up again for another year. Told you, I'm not proud. Eventually my doctor and wife both figured out what I did, so back on the schedule I went. While I was waiting, I had a small outpatient procedure done that required knocking me out. Afterward the anesthesiologist came to check up on me. "I noticed something while you were out. Have you ever been evaluated for sleep apnea?" she asked. Before I could even open my mouth, my wife interjected, "His sleep study is next week," then turned to me with a crooked smile.

Yes, dear.

The sleep study was not the best night I've ever spent away from home, to be sure, but it also wasn't that bad. And sure enough, about 2:30 a.m., on went the Vader mask. Another diagnosis. Great.

In only a few days I had my own CPAP machine, which I affectionately call the *Infernal Contraption*, that sits next to my side of the bed. It has got a long hose, makes surprisingly little noise, and will automatically phone home with each night's sleep results. It is a little creepy if you think about it, so I don't. For some, the CPAP is a life-changing thing. Finally sleeping well means people discover rest and energy they didn't know they had. Some report remarkable increases in their ability to concentrate and the need for daily naps disappears. While I doubt anyone will be asking for my testimonial anytime soon, I must confess it helps. Nights I cannot wear it I feel it the next day to be sure. Turns out I really was not sleeping well before, and now I am. Plus, as a bonus, my heart was not spending its sleeping hours beating like a meth-addicted monkey. So that's good.

Nobody knows how many midlife heart attacks are related to undiagnosed sleep apnea, but it's no doubt a lot. In my wife's practice, almost everyone gets a sleep study, especially if they are looking for help with weight loss. A tired body does not process food well and a tired mind does not make good decisions. The rates in the US for sleep apnea have increased dramatically over the last few years, but it is not known if that is happening because more people have it or if more common testing means previously undiagnosed people are now getting diagnosed. Likely a mixture of both.

To be clear, my CPAP has joined the list of things I don't like but recognize I must do, that also includes my injected medication and regular blood draws. At first I didn't bring my CPAP with me when I traveled but I recognized that was not a good plan. So now I bring it with me. The nice part is nearly every airline will let you bring it on as an additional carryon for no extra charge. The bad thing is, in a time when checked baggage fees mean everyone carries on all they can, other people don't know that. I was once waiting at the front of the line for group three, waiting to board my plane home. I had my regulation-sized roller bag in one hand, my CPAP bag perched on top, and my backpack over my shoulder. Like most people I was tuning out the announcements about this being a very full flight and some people would need to check a bag or two. Maybe those poor schmoes in group five, but I was in three, and in the front of the line, no less. As I waited I started to tune in to the conversation happening near the front of the group four line. Somebody was complaining to a friend about the guy trying to get onboard with too much stuff. *Yeah, screw that guy,* I thought. As I looked around I caught the eye of the person I suspected was doing the complaining. When he looked back at me I very quickly realized what I had missed before: I was *that guy.* Turn around, I thought, and look at the floor. Thankfully group two was just then called and within minutes I was up at the boarding gate. As the gate agent scanned my ticket and I walked through the doors I heard a not so subtle, "What the hell!" from a familiar-sounding voice. As I walked down the Jetway I simply prayed, "Please, God, let him be seated somewhere in front of me, not behind me."

When I travel for work now it is often with the same people, and I am grateful that my typical roommate on these trips has not been bothered by the Infernal Contraption. To be honest, it is embarrassing to use or talk about. For years I knew they were common among older people, but I was in my late thirties. Was I really going to spend my nights for the next forty years hooked up to this thing, or was the universe just trying to tell me, *forty more years might be a little ambitious.* The cold reality is that the average life expectancy is for the first time no longer increasing in the US, and in some measures actually decreasing. From where I sit, it is no wonder why.

So sleeping is now added to the list of basic biological functions my body doesn't do well, along with processing sugar, the basic fuel it runs on. You start to wonder what you might have done wrong in a previous life to deserve all this and how things could get any worse. That last part, obviously, you don't want an answer to. Unfortunately, I got one.

I am going to warn you this next part is about sex. If you don't want to read it, that is fine, skip ahead to where you see the ***.

So I am a guy, and like most guys there is another basic biological function I rather enjoy. Bonus, as a married guy, I have someone who lives in my house to enjoy it with. Assuming, of course, she's feeling into it. I personally don't think there is anything wrong with liking sex. I also firmly believe sex is something God gave us to enjoy, so we shouldn't feel guilty or weird about enjoying it. That said, I also think sex is special and is something that binds two people together, so we need to be careful how we practice it. None of that is really the point of this part, however, except to say that I think a healthy, respectful sex life is an important part of a healthy, respectful relationship.

Sex is already intertwined deeply with things like body image and self-worth, so anything that complicates things further is truly unwanted.

As stated way back in the beginning of this book, diabetes is a cardiovascular condition. Meaning, it effects your blood, your veins, and everywhere you blood goes. For men there is one place your blood goes that feels pretty important. Unlike some other animals, humans have no penis bone. While other primates have some extra help down there, human males are left with blood flow, and blood flow alone, to keep erect during sex. When you're young this is no big deal. Combine the natural onset of middle age with a chronic medical condition that affects your veins and blood flow, and it can become a pretty big deal.

Most marriages run on routine. I do the dishes and my wife the laundry. Sometimes we may bicker about which is the larger job, but I know a sink full of dirty plates is my cue. I am actually a big fan of routine. I like know what to expect. It is the same when it comes to sex. Don't get me wrong; I don't mind it if we spice it up now and then. But I also appreciate what is comfortable and familiar. One great gift of a long-term relationship is that you learn what your partner likes. It lowers the anxiety when you know going in what generally your partner appreciates and what they don't.

While many jokes have been made about Viagra and similar drugs, they are attempting to address a very real problem. Erectile dysfunction (ED for short) is, first off, a terrible name. I am not sure what would be better, but I am not a fan. ED is also sneaky. You may start out feeling fine and up for the task at hand only to figure out later, things aren't quite right. The old adage is true: *it does happen to every guy*. Once in a great while and usually for a reason. What I started to experience was happening more often than could be easily be dismissed, and for no obvious reason. Previously predictably pleasurable routines seemed to be suddenly not so predictable. What would start out as a fun evening would end up in a place of frustration and angst. Most often we would get through warm up fine and issues would not arise until we were well into the main event. Then everything would just sort of shut down physically. This had no effect on anything else, so of course my brain would still be screaming for climax while my body was simply unable to comply. My wife, being the generous person she is, would offer no end of, "It's okay" and, "We can take a break for a moment," but nothing really helped. Sometimes I could tell trouble was coming, but like an oncoming train, there was nothing I could do to stop it.

I may not enjoy talking to my doctor about my diabetes, my sleeping, or any of the rest of it. This one, however, this one I would talk about. Not because I wanted to, mind you, but this was just that important. I actually ended up talking to the

NP who worked with my doctor, and I was fine with that. We talked through the options, the different drugs, and how they worked. She even reviewed with me the importance of foreplay for both of us. It was a very professional and matter-of-fact conversation that somehow felt almost normal. I am not sure if I was just getting used to discussing personal details in exam rooms, but I found myself talking about things I would never mention outside of one. As I write this I am not sure this section will actually make it in the final draft or if modesty will overcome me and I will pull it out. If you are reading, I guess you know the answer.

Perhaps what really tipped the scales was that this was something I could not hide. It is not that I hide things from my wife on purpose, but I do sometimes fail to share things I don't really want to talk about. There was no way to cover up this one. She knew as well as I that all was not well. Sometimes just one other person knowing you are struggling can make the difference. Not just with ED, but with all sorts of things. There is a big difference between feeling alone and not feeling alone, and the second is always better.

***

Both the infernal contraption and my new blue pills are a sign of something I always knew but tried to ignore: diabetes is a progressive condition, meaning that it doesn't stand still. Your medication routine might work now but not next year. You may have ten eye exams in a row that are fine, but on the eleventh, *Houston, we have a problem.* The condition is dynamic; it shifts and changes because you are shifting and changing. Sometimes I think we have this idea that our bodies grow and change when we are young, then stay pretty much the same for a while until we get old and then they decline quickly. Unfortunately that is not true. In response to how you eat, sleep, exercise, and the season, your body is always changing. Sometimes for the better, sometimes not. No matter what, it is a moving target.

I am someone who likes some variety in life. I gave a presentation about the work my church had done in the community after I had been there about three years. It was impressive what we had managed to accomplish together. After I was done I was chatting with someone I knew only in passing. She asked, "What you've done at the church all sounds great. So, you bored yet?" I hadn't thought about it really, but if I was honest, yeah, I was getting a little bored. So it is not like I am against things changing. In fact, I kind of like it. One way I accommodate the change I want to see is to minimize change in any other way. I have threatened my wife that I might go full Steve Jobs one day and just adopt a standard outfit and buy a dozen copies. She's not keen on the idea. Like most people, I want my diabetes firmly in the consistency column. All the medication, finger sticks, and diet restrictions are bad enough without needing to change them too often.

It is hard enough to navigate the world when you already feel like there is so much going against you. When you do find a routine that is not contributing to the possibility of an early demise, it sucks beyond compare when the sand shifts under your feet. If you are dealing with that sort of thing, I sympathize. Nobody likes a moving target. All I can say is that you will find a new normal if you keep looking. It's not fair, to be sure, but we humans are very adaptable. Keep with it. Drugs will come and go, diets will come and go, routines will come and go. What stays the same is the basic fact that despite all the challenges it comes with, life is a gift that we all deserve to enjoy as long as possible.

9. Changing Times

I can give pretty much anybody the benefit of the doubt. I know I am not perfect, and I say and do things that hurt people. Most of the time I don't mean to and a good chunk of the time I am actually trying to help. So when others do or say things that I find hurtful I do my best to let it go and recognize their intentions first and foremost. This is all part of embracing brokenness. Sometimes my brokenness shows to others in ways I wish it didn't, so I cannot be surprised when theirs shows, too. This is, at least, what I try to do. Sometimes, though, it feels impossible.

Early in the process of writing this book, somewhere around drafting chapter two, I got a call from a friend asking if we could talk. He was going through some difficult things with his marriage and needed a friendly ear. We agreed to meet an hour later at a local coffee shop. A trip out of the house was fine with me, and I try to help where I can. I arrived first, ordered my dirty hot chai tea, and waited. As I stood there, waiting for my drink, the barista was talking to the person who ordered in front of me. He was speaking in such a way that it was obvious he didn't mind me overhearing his conversation, though in the beginning, I tried not to. What perked my interest is when I heard the word *pastor*. I live my life surrounded by church people who talk about church things. I am, after all, a pastor. But when I am out in the rest of the world I don't usually expect to hear church talk. So, I started to tune in to what the guy making my coffee was saying. I don't know what led him to the point he was at, but by the time I started listening he was going on about how overweight pastors are inappropriate. Further, he alluded to the fact that being overweight might even be sinful.

I swear to God that really happened.

Here I am writing a book that is about the difficult realities of having diabetes in America today and the associated weight issues that often go with it, and this guy is going off about how I, as both a pastor and an overweight person, might be flaunting my sin. I literally had no words. I knew I needed to be fully present for my friend who was coming shortly so I decided not to engage with the guy. My friend was coming to me for help, so finding me in a heated theological debate with the coffee shop staff probably would not be appropriate.

Let me just say this to all of you reading very clearly. I can typically understand where people are coming from, theologically speaking, even if I don't agree with them. I have read my Bible cover to cover, studied it along with many great Christian thinkers. Heck, I have a master's degree in it and years of practice standing in front of people weekly explaining faith, scripture, and God's desires for our lives. I have developed daily routines I believe help me keep in tune with the movements of the Holy Spirit, and I pray, often. I am by no means the greatest at any of these things, sometimes I am actually pretty lousy at them, but I am not just some guy off the street either.

So with all that in mind, let me just say this. I have no clue where this guy was coming from. The heart of the biblical message is that we are all created in God's image, we call it the *imago Dei*. Being created in God's image is not about how we look on the outside; it is on the inside where we find the likeness. We are in God's image because we love, celebrate, and mourn. We experience loss because we are in God's image, and we experience joy for the same reason. When asked what the most important teaching of all the scripture was, Jesus replied, "'Love the Lord your God with all your heart and with all your soul and with all your strength and with all your mind'; and, 'Love your neighbor as yourself.'" That ability to show and receive love, that is the image of God.

My faith tells me God intends people to come in all shapes, sizes, and colors. Diversity is part of the plan. The only place God asks for uniformity is in how we love; in everything else, diversity is the goal. Yes, the early Christian writer Paul did say, "There is neither Jew nor Gentile, neither slave nor free, nor is there male and female, for you are all one in Christ Jesus," but he never meant to say that these distinctions would disappear. He meant we are supposed to stop using them as ways of separating ourselves from one another. God creates a diversity of people on the outside with the same capacity for love on the inside. For my money you can add "neither skinny nor fat" to Paul's list.

The barista's thinking is not only wrong, it is dangerous. It can feed all the destructive cycles of shame and guilt I know so well. I take some comfort in the fact that this line of thinking is not one I commonly find in the church, though I fear it is far more common in the rest of the world than we would like to believe.

One place my driver's license gave me access to growing up was Dairy Queen, a place my friends and I would go often. As much as I like soft-serve ice cream, that was not the reason for going. The reason we went was that the DQ is where all the cute girls worked. No joke, and I don't believe that was just a coincidence. If you are an employer you are not allowed to base your hiring or firing on things like race, gender, or age. You are, however, allowed to decide whatever you want on the basis of appearance and whatever you decide that appearance means. And this happens all the time.

The bias gets repeated up the economic food chain as far as you care to go. An experiment was done by a pair of researchers that showed candidates' resumes and pictures to corporate hiring professionals. In their study they uncovered a strong bias against overweight people. Candidates with an obese appearance, but identical resumes to skinny candidates, were consistently rated as seeming less competent than their skinnier counterparts. Some might point to this widespread, almost unconscious, bias as proof that there is something to the idea that being overweight is somehow intrinsically a bad thing. Well, hold on a minute. Let me tell you a story.

I am not much of an art fan but I love history. During that same summer in Germany that I discovered Germans' odd proclivities about soda, my future wife joined me for a couple weeks to relieve my feeling of isolation. Since she was there we decided to spend a weekend in Rome and look at old stuff. We saw the Colosseum, the Pantheon, and took a tour of the Vatican. This was before I had any renewed interest in church but it was still interesting. The Vatican is full of art. Like, full! Over the centuries they were patrons to all sorts of artisans and their work is around today as a legacy.

Most of what you see on display is centuries old and some even older.

As we walked the hallways taking it all in, I started to notice something. Many of the people depicted in the pictures seemed different than what you'd expect to see today. Especially the nudes. It took me a while to put my finger on it but eventually I clued in to something. Most of the women in the paintings we were seeing would be a size twelve to sixteen in contemporary sizes. That is enough to warrant getting booted out of the regular-size clothing section of most department stores into the plus-size area. What was going on? Given the poses and context of the people being depicted in the paintings, these were not just portraits of people who happened to be a little bigger, but instead they were intended to be representations of concepts like beauty and attractiveness. To see what I am on about, look no further than Renaissance era depictions of Adam and Eve (Tiziano Vecellio's is a favorite of mine). Adam is often depicted trim and toned as you'd expect, but Eve invariably has full hips, a bit of a tummy, and small breasts. There is no thigh gap to be found within a hundred miles of any of these pictures. And this is Eve, the godly ideal of womanhood.

The truth is, where and when we live shapes our understanding of beauty more than we might expect. In the days of the Middle Ages and into the Renaissance, nearly everyone was involved in one

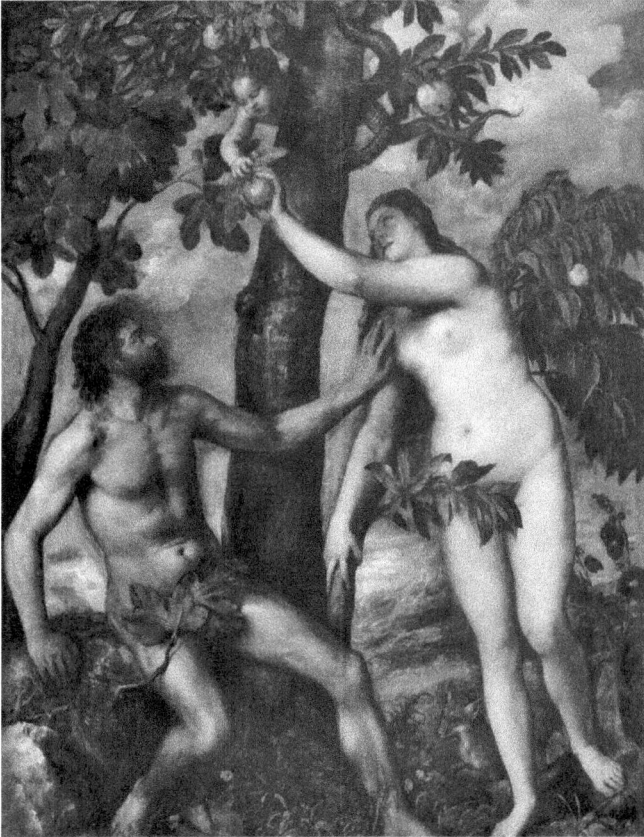

The Fall of Man by Tiziano Vecellio

way or another in the growing of food. Cultivating fields is very hard work when you have no tractor or other machines to help you. Nearly everyone lived in rural communities, walked everywhere, and had access to only enough calories to survive. It was just the wealthy or noble, the equivalent to the contemporary 1 percent, who had access to enough food on a regular enough basis to have a BMI north of twenty-five. So being bigger was a sign not of failure but success. It meant you could afford to labor less and eat more than nearly everyone else. This is also why both the men and women in these portraits are so pale. Only those who didn't work in fields all day could be so lightly tinted. I had previously wondered why portraits of old kings seemed to almost celebrate their girth. Google a picture of Henry VIII to see what I mean. Now it makes perfect sense.

The modern notion that we are supposed to be skinny and tan to be considered attractive exists for the same reason it used to be the reverse; it is a sign of prosperity. Gym memberships, tanning salons, and fresh organic food all cost money that not everyone can afford. The Renaissance equivalent of my barista friend would have likely complained about priests who were too skinny. *Shouldn't they be demonstrating the abundant love of Christ and the power of the church through their ample appearance?* Have another piece of cake, Friar!

Knowing that what constitutes a desirable appearance is mostly made up helps, somewhat. It is nice to know that my current above average BMI means someone who looks like me would be exactly what all the ladies were into 400 years ago. But people also regularly died of gingivitis back then, too (not kidding), so I will keep the twenty-first century, thanks. When we talk about body image we often do it in relation to the messages media is sending to young girls, and that is important. We should worry about that. What I am guessing most people don't know is that men and young boys are concerned about their appearances, too. That fact is not so well discussed.

We all carry excess weight in slightly different ways on our bodies. Some people carry their extra pounds on their hips and thighs. For others it is more around the middle. I am a man who carries some of that extra weight in the chest area. There is no fact about myself I hate, and I mean *hate*, more than that.

This has been the case my whole life, which meant shower time in high-school gym class was akin to getting a tooth extracted on a daily basis. It was honestly torture. Adolescents are not well known for their sensitivity to the feelings of others. This is actually biological because that part of their brains isn't fully developed yet. Which means, God help anyone who stands out in any way. I heard every snicker and perceived every sideways look. Once, when forced into a game of shirts and skins in the main gym, I seriously considered faking an ankle injury. As the gym filled with people from other classes, I felt physically ill. Even today you will more likely find me next to a pool with my shirt on than in the pool with it off. All of this informs how I feel about myself on a regular basis, and none of it is anything I am likely to share with others. I know diet and exercise are the way out, but even if my body suddenly changed tomorrow, all the experiences I have had over the years are still in my head and not going anywhere.

Keen observers will note that the exercise part of *diet and exercise* hasn't featured that much in this book. That is true. That is because it doesn't feature much in my life. Activity level in America has charted a similar course to diet in a lot of ways. While we have greater access to high-sugar and high-fat food than ever before, we also have greater access to low-activity jobs and entertainment than ever before. Video games have long since replaced pickup basketball games for young people. And before you start going all, *those darn kids today!* you should really be more worried about *those darn adults today!*

Not long ago more people lived in rural areas than in cities because most of them were involved in one of two things: growing food or making things. Both of these jobs require physical labor, and the idea that you needed to add additional exercise on top of that was unheard of. Today, as more people live in cities and our economy is dominated by office and service work, things are different. The standing-desk fad was one way to address the fact that more and more of us spend our days in front computer screens and sitting in chairs. It is becoming increasingly clear our bodies were not meant to do this much sitting. My back will remind me of that if I push it too long.

We can no longer take for granted that we will naturally get the amount of physical activity our bodies need. Instead we are expected to go to the gym, go for runs, or otherwise add high-exertion activities to our days to fill the gap. And we *should* do this. But we should also not be surprised that it is difficult to do. Most Americans actually work more than forty hours a week, and overall Americans work more hours a week than any other comparable country. Stagnant wage growth also means people are increasingly working multiple jobs to make ends meet. Add in family commitments, and even getting thirty minutes of exercise a day is a big challenge for most.

The plain truth is that we have created a situation in our country where many people simply cannot afford to be healthy. I don't want to take all the pills I take to treat my diabetes; I also know that getting more exercise would make it more likely I could take less, but we shouldn't pretend that is an easy thing to do. I am actually lucky in the fact that I have not one but two gym memberships, one of which is only a couple blocks from my office. I often wonder what people who are not as lucky as I am are supposed to do?

There is a cost for our drive for ever greater productivity. We may be one of the most innovative and productive countries in the world, but let's not pretend that didn't come with some trade-offs. One of two things is true. Either we have lost all sense of self-control when it comes to food and activity level, which is why obesity and diabetes are on the rise, or we are all attempting to navigate an unprecedented situation of abundant high-calorie food and very low daily physical demands. Obviously I think it is the latter. For a long time, replacing physical labor on farms and in factories with machines was considered progress. It gave us access to lots of cheap food and products. We are now discovering the consequences that come with all the progress. We continue to inhabit bodies that are designed to run on far less fuel and do far harder work than most of us will ever need to ask them to do. So we shouldn't be surprised when complications arise.

The barista from the beginning of the chapter didn't mean to set something off inside of me, but he did. Living with diabetes can feel like living in a minefield. Some of the mines are obvious, and some are not. When you have diabetes, you are also forced to either invite people into your minefield or live without the types of close relationships everyone craves. One day I had a particularly bad blood sugar reading on my morning test that I could not explain. I was getting down on myself in the shower and as I dressed. By time I emerged from the bedroom in search of my morning coffee I was in a full-on *mood*. I am not sure what my wife even said to me but I lashed out in return. I had been standing with my toe on a mine and she just kicked it over. It was not her fault. Even as it was happening, I knew that. I also could not really explain it to her because I was not entirely certain myself how I arrived at such a negative place. She left for work angry, and I spent my day feeling very low. I don't want to subject those I love to my minefield, but it feels like it is an unavoidable part of hanging around me. The world demands that I exercise more self-control than I feel I can muster most of the time. That drains my energy before I even start working on all the rest of my responsibilities like work and family.

Even those who mean well can sometimes be the exact opposite of what you need. Shortly after my diagnosis I was attending a family dinner at my grandparents' house. It was a nice time until dessert came around. My mother had brought angel food cake and strawberry topping. I was trying to be good about diet so I declined. Unfortunately my mother persisted and insisted it was fine and that I could have some despite knowing about my condition, forcing me into eating it or making a scene. Looking back, I appreciate she worked hard making it and wanted us to enjoy it, but at the same time, don't I get to decide what's okay and what is not for me to eat?

If you are reading this book because someone you care about has diabetes, I am grateful you are. The more you know, the more supportive you can be, and your friend or loved one needs your support. However, I need to be clear about what that support looks like. Nearly everyone with diabetes has a small army of medical providers, nutritionists, and educators at their disposal. I regularly get calls from diabetes experts who work for my insurance company, ready and willing to help me understand anything I need to know. They have a vested interest, after all, in seeing me go to the gym more and the pharmacy less. All of us have ready access to experts. We don't need more experts. We need friends.

What I crave from my close friends and family is people who will listen without judging. I need them to hear my problems without trying to solve them. After a long day, when I order dessert at that special restaurant I love, I need them to grab a spoon and dig in with me, not shoot me disappointed looks. And when I do manage to get my sorry butt to the gym, lay off the pasta, and maybe even drop a couple A1c percentage points, I need them to celebrate with me and recognize how big a deal that is. Since so few of us talk about our condition at all, that means when the successes do come, we often celebrate alone.

Finally, please recognize that we are more than our condition. I used to say that *I am diabetic*. I thought it sounded better than *I have diabetes*, because I cannot hear the word *diabetes* without hearing it in Wilford Brimley's voice (no disrespect intended, Mr. Brimley). The problem is that I am not diabetic. Of course, I do have diabetes, but I am not diabetic in the same way that I am a husband, a father, or a Christian. I don't need or want my condition to define me. It is not who I am; it is a condition I have. This book has been about one part of my life, but it is just that, one part. I am so much more than that. So your friend or loved one needs you to know that, too. Some days having diabetes is the biggest thing in your life; most days it is not.

If you are reading this and you are the one with diabetes, you need to know this more than anything. Your condition does not define you: you are so much more. Yes, do the finger sticks, take the drugs, refill the insulin pump, then get on with all the other far more important things you need to do. Because you are far more complex, interesting, and dynamic than any one line in your medical chart. Remember that above all else.

10. Don't Go It Alone

Back when I first started to attend church and work with the youth group, I was invited to be part of another kind of group. Several of the youth leaders from different churches in the area had become friends. They formed a Thursday lunch group that I was invited to join. It was mostly a time to chat, share, and enjoy each other's company. Even just that, in a world addicted to moving ever faster, is a treat. Café culture in places like Italy and France still supports these types of encounters, and I think that is something we miss out on. It has been amazing to me how many different coffee circles I have noticed older people get involved in when they retire. Relieved of the daily burden of work, it is like they all wake up and remember that being around other people is a good thing.

Our Thursday group had a slightly deeper level to it than just conversation. We called it our *accountability group.* It was intended to be a time we could share about what was really going on in our lives and find support. Not "fixing things" sort of support, but a true listening sort of support. Sometimes all you really need is to feel honestly listened to. Saying things out loud, knowing other people are aware of what's going on in the shadows of your life, can give you a sort of strength. It breaks feelings of isolation, and when you have to put your problems into words, you often realize they are not as big as they seemed in your head. It can also make practicing the massive amount of self-control required in today's world a little easier.

It's not that I expected them to call me out if they heard of me doing something I was trying not to. Just them knowing, feeling like others were aware and supportive, was often enough to give my self-control a boost. Too often we believe there must be negative consequences if we want people to change their behavior. Perhaps. But we shouldn't overlook the power of others simply being aware. Honestly, if I give in to something I shouldn't, I will beat myself up enough for it, I promise. I don't really need my friends joining in with that part. Our group was not always perfect. Sometimes the conversation stayed very shallow. But sometimes, when it was needed, we could be there for each other in a way few people are.

Moving to Ohio, one thing I feared I would miss is my small group, but that fear turned out to be unfounded. Through providence or dumb luck, a fellow student I befriended in the first couple weeks on campus shared he was looking to start a similar group. We drafted in another guy and for the next two years, every Thursday night, we gathered for a couple hours, after the kids were all in bed, to discuss school, family, life, and whatever else was on our hearts. It is amazing how quickly in these situations people will start to open up. Some part of us craves this kind of deep community, and when we encounter it, the floodgates open. We discovered we had similar challenges and fears. When I was afraid of losing my scholarship after my first-semester grades were below the minimum required, these are the guys I worked that through with. We talked about our marriages, our dreams, and our fears. There are so many stories I wish I could tell you, but these groups are also highly confidential, so I honestly cannot.

Folks who lived in the building we would meet in started to call us the *three wise men*. I am not sure we were all that wise, but I will say that being part of that group was one of the best decisions I made when I was there. The group changed after two years as members started graduating. In the four years I was in school the composition of the group changed several times, but I always tried to keep it going. I needed it. Sometimes other folks would try to find their way in and I would suggest they start their own group instead. Three is just a good number for this type of thing.

When I left school and moved back to Montana with my family to be a pastor, it took me a long time to find something similar to what I had before. It took years, in fact. While pastors in our area were organized into small groups called clusters, the intention of these groups seemed different than what I had known before. Not bad, just different. I came to a place where I missed having regular, deep conversation with others. Being a pastor can be an isolating job. People typically only reach out to you if there is some sort of crisis or they need something. You have to be careful where you let your guard down because what you say and do carries weight. I quickly realized my tendency to think out loud was going to get me into trouble. Offhand comments I made circulated through the church rumor mill and would come back to me in a much more interesting form.

About two years into living in Montana, I attended a conference in Denver, Colorado, with some fellow pastors. We drove, so we had lots of time to chat on the way back. It was here I discovered I was not the only one looking for a deeper type of community, and by the time we hit the border, we had arranged to start an online group that would meet weekly over video chat. That has been happening on and off ever since.

At one time, humans almost all lived in smaller villages with no TVs to entertain us. Houses were small, and you would not spend very much time in them. For the last couple of years in Ohio, we lived on a street where the houses were older and the front of them all lined up so you could see from your large front porch all the way down the block across all the other front porches. In my time there, those porches were almost always empty, but I imagine there was a time when that was not true and they were full of life. After all, why build them if you didn't plan on using them? When we lived in Albuquerque we got to know our neighbors on one side of us. She was from Mexico, and he was from Scotland. They both worked at the local university in the international studies department, of course. During one conversation, our Scottish neighbor shared that when they first moved in he was in love with his garage. He really enjoyed that you could pull your car right in then go straight inside. Lately, though, he was reconsidering. Where he had lived in Scotland everybody parked on the street, so when you got home and moved from your car to your house you had the opportunity to interact with people. He missed that. In fact, we had only met after encountering each other at the large communal mailboxes, which was the only place people in our neighborhood congregated. And this happened after we had lived only feet apart for months. Technology like smartphones and Facebook has gotten a lot of blame for creating a greater sense of disconnectedness in society today. Perhaps that is true. But we cannot overlook other things that are contributing, like the ever-increasing average home size. We have larger homes that we are spending more and more time in. Perhaps that is why younger people are actually leaving the suburbs and heading back into urban city centers in droves. Proximity to communal space like Starbucks is more of a priority than large amounts of personal living space. They are trying to reclaim something their parents and grandparents left behind.

Feeling isolated is not just something that gets you down or makes life less fun; it is far more serious than that. A recent study showed that being isolated from others can actually increase your risk of a heart attack by 29 percent and a stroke by 32 percent. A survey by AARP of older adults showed rates of loneliness had doubled from 20 percent to 40 percent in recent years. Humans are by nature communal. We prefer to run in packs, much like wolves, and it has been that way since the beginning. We don't generally respond well to feeling alone or isolated. When these natural desires for community are complicated by having a condition like diabetes, things get even harder to navigate.

In many ways Starbucks and its many copycats are bringing back café culture in the United States, and I think that is a good thing. I have most meetings now not in my office but in various coffee shops and restaurants all over town. The challenge is that most drink options you find at these places have enough sugar in them to orbit a small dog. It is not that I cannot order a black coffee; of course I can. But meeting in places like these means I have to actively resist the caramel macchiato I really want, and it is oftentimes easier to just not come inside than make that choice. Meeting people socially in places that serve food and drinks when you have diabetes means mentally preparing yourself to practice an extra level of self-control. Being social in these situations can actually make you feel *more* isolated, not less. And as already stated, feeling isolated is not a good thing.

I started the project that became this book for a simple reason: to tell a true story about what it is like to have diabetes in America today. Along the way, as I researched and developed my outlines and drafts, it became more than that. What I discovered is how much things have changed and how quickly. I grew up dazzled at how we were exploring the outer reaches of our solar system. I marveled at the first real picture of Pluto sent back by NASA's New Horizons probe. I have seen cars get faster, safer, and more like spaceships full of touchscreens and automatic braking. I went from my first Mac Plus computer to the crazy capable MacBook Pro I am typing on right now. Progress is all around us all the time. This part of the story is well told. What I have found is not so well told is the other side of the story. It seems painfully obvious to me now that our lives are changing far faster than our bodies can keep up with.

Through the millennia, up until only a few decades ago, our bodies needed to store every extra bit of energy they could, because famine could always be just around the corner. Our amazing ability to eat both meat and plants meant we could adapt and thrive in ways no other animal could. It made us the top dogs anyplace we went and allowed us to cover the globe. This amazing ability of the human body is, very unfortunately, still being put to use today in the poorest parts of our world where food is still scarce. Starvation has not been eradicated; far from it.

In the part of the world I live in, safe within the borders of the richest, most powerful nation the world has ever seen, things are different. Our bodies are not adapted yet to a life where food is abundant and demands for physical labor are low. What took centuries to develop in us is not going to change overnight. So whether we want to be or not, we are stuck where we are. I am not arguing for giving up the advances in agriculture that have put the eradication of hunger within our reach. I don't want to scavenge for food, and I am glad robots have taken over the dirtiest and most dangerous jobs in our factories. That is truly progress. That progress, however, has come at a price, one that we are only now starting to understand.

I am convinced the epidemic of diabetes that is sweeping across the world is simply a logical byproduct of the contemporary world we are living in. Our bodies are attempting to overcome previously unknown challenges, and we are finding the weaknesses in our design. Our bodies have never had the ability to deal with the levels of sugar or inactivity that are common today, but they have also never been asked to try to bear them before. Because we are diverse creatures, some of us are faring better than others. That is good. If you are one of the lucky ones who is successfully navigating all there is to tempt us today, I am glad for that. Frankly you give me hope that we will find a way through the maze of unintended consequences we find ourselves in. I ask just one thing: don't look down on us who are struggling. Trust me, we know when we fail. If you find it easy to move through the abundant unhealthy choices we all face, great; just don't expect it to be as easy for everyone. After all, it is not actually possible to walk a mile in any shoes but your own, so we shouldn't pretend we truly know what others are going through.

For you, my fellow travelers on the diabetes road, I hope you know one thing: you are not alone. For some reason each of us has been born into a moment of history where we get to witness great change. I don't know what this period will be called, but like the Renaissance or industrial revolution, I am certain history will give it a name. I like my smartphone and high-speed internet, and I cannot wait for a car that drives itself. I don't want to live in any other time than this. I am excited to be one of the many who have moved back into a downtown area where house lots might be small but neighborhoods feel more alive. I cannot wait to see what is around the corner and what the next must-have killer app will be. This is truly a good time to be alive.

At the same time, I am fully aware of the challenges contemporary life brings to me as a person with diabetes. I reject the idea that this is all simply my fault for not having enough self-control. When companies worth billions of dollars spend millions of those dollars each year on marketing and advertising to convince me to buy products that are dangerous to my health, that is not just about me and my issues. When I was seven or eight I got drenched in a backyard water fight. I left everything I had in my pockets on the side porch to dry, including a couple five-dollar bills. Later I opened the door just in time to see the neighbor boy lifting one. Yeah, he had some blame in that, but so did I. Recently I took my car in to be serviced and there was a sign on the wall reminding you to take your valuables with you and in big letters on top read, "Thou Shall Not Tempt," advice our current culture is thoroughly ignoring. People's livelihoods are dependent on convincing you that eating an individually wrapped fruit pie packed with 60-plus grams of sugar is an okay thing to do. Further, these are nice people with families and friends who depend on them. There are no white hats and black hats in this struggle. We are all in it together.

The plain truth is that having diabetes sucks and it brings with it a whole lot of work most people would rather not do. Myself included. Unfortunately the work must be done. Knowing all I know now actually helps and gives me some hope. For a while it felt like it was me alone against the world, and I now realize that is not true. Yes, the world may actually be against me sometimes, but I am never alone. There are so many other people out there who are dealing with the same things I am.

I wish I could end this by telling you the story of my personal triumph over diabetes, but I cannot. I am still working on it one day at a time, some days being better than others. The best news I have had recently is when I replaced my blood meter. Turns out that the old one was constantly reading 30 points too high. Check your equipment, people! Honestly, even though it didn't really change anything, it felt like a victory. Here I was, writing this book, and I could not get my morning test into my goal range. Turns out it was actually fine.

I pray you have found some comfort and hope in these pages. I never intended to give you excuses but instead motivation. We need to name the truth of what is going on if we are to work through it. There is a quote from Jesus in the Bible I feel I understand better now. It goes like this: "Suppose one of you wants to build a tower. Won't you first sit down and estimate the cost to see if you have enough money to complete it?" We each have a tower to build, which is our lives. It is critical to talk honestly about the challenges we will face building it. Now that you have a better understanding about what you are up against, where do you start? Well, same as with any tower, one brick at a time. Things won't be perfect tomorrow. You won't find a deep and abiding love of Brussels sprouts at your next meal. That's okay. Just do all you can tomorrow to make it a little better. The gift and curse of having diabetes is that it is a slowly developing condition. That means you have time. Time to ignore it, or time to improve it. That, my friend, is your real choice. I believe in myself, and I believe in you. Two steps forward and one step back will eventually get you there, so have some grace with yourself on the backward steps. They happen to all of us.

If you reached the end of this book and you read it alone, let me suggest this. The most successful Las Vegas card counters in history were a group of MIT students who played as a team. As you play your hand against the stacked deck, don't do it alone. Find folks you can trust and sit down at the same playing table as them. Maybe read this book together. Because we know one thing for sure: when two or more start working together to play against the house, the odds change!

God bless you on your journey.

A. Small Group Reading Guide

Reading this book as a small group can give you the opportunity to invite those close to you into an important conversation. Reading the book gives the group a common experience to discuss and provides those who might relate to sections of it a way to share what they are feeling. Not everyone will agree on all points, and that is okay. Some might not even like the book, that's okay too. The point is to create an opportunity for people to share what is on their minds.

Other chronic medical conditions exist, like heart disease, asthma, arthritis, osteoporosis, and others. While those conditions are not the subject of this book, they come with similar challenges. Don't limit your group to just those affected by diabetes. This is a good way to start a wider conversation about chronic health conditions as a whole.

Who is in the group?

Who you invite to read this book with you is up to you, but be mindful of a couple of things. First, the actual point of a discussion group is, well, discussion. The conversation that happens between people, and relationships that form or deepen because of it, are what you are after. So make sure the people you invite are interested and willing to be in conversation.

Second, confidentiality is important. Some people will open up quickly in a small group setting and are willing to share very honestly. Everyone should respect that and hold whatever is said in confidence. Your aim is to build trust and nothing will destroy trust faster than breaking confidentiality.

Group dynamics change if the group gets bigger than nine or so people. Over that size it is too easy for quieter people to get lost and for more talkative people to dominate. Best to keep the group small.

Setting a time and place

Some book clubs, for example, meet monthly and discuss an entire book. This particular book would be better discussed one or two chapters at a time over the course of several weekly sessions. This is a larger commitment, of course, but it will definitely lead to a better experience.

Find a place that is comfortable and accessible to all. Public places like diners or coffee shops can work so long as everyone can actually hear each other. Some places have the music turned up so loud it's impossible to understand what others are saying.

Time of day should be based on whatever is convenient for the group. Don't overlook the lunch hour, which will have the bonus of keeping you from running too long. Whenever you meet, you will need to respect that people are busy and some folks will not be able to linger beyond an hour or so.

The gatherings

The gatherings of your group can be as simple or complex as you like. They can be as easy as asking people in turn, "What did you take away most from this chapter(s)?" then allowing the conversation to unfold naturally. Just make sure everyone gets a chance to answer.

It is always good to end with a time of mutual sharing and support. This also can be as simple as asking each person, "What can we be praying/thinking/meditating about for you this coming week?" Again, just make sure everyone has the opportunity to answer.

Some groups may want to add singing, sacred text reading, or other elements, depending on who is in the group. That is fine. In the beginning, whatever you do will feel a little forced, but quickly it will become natural. Just stick with it and have fun. If you are doing it right, it should quickly stop feeling artificial and instead become something you look forward to doing.

B. Note to Health-care Professionals
By Daen Scott APRN, FNP-BC, CDE

The American Diabetes Association Standards of Care contains an entire section reminding us to keep an eye not just on labs but on the psychosocial health of our patients. It's all too easy to get caught up in numbers on a page and forget the day-to-day burden chronic issues like diabetes place on the person sitting across from us.

In reading this book or in recommending it to your patients, I would urge you to use it as a tool to move the conversation from, "How do we work with diabetic patients?" to, "How do we work with people who have diabetes?" The difference may seem semantic, but there's a reason the ADA is pushing to avoid using the former term in reference to people. The human beings we treat are much more than their A1c's, and we have to make them partners in their own care. All the prescriptions in the world won't help if the person doesn't have the tools, the knowledge, and the buy-in to make the day-to-day choices that create health.

Jeremy mentions early in the book that I tell my patients, "Diabetes is the hobby no one wants." This is true. And I will assert that many of my most challenging, "noncompliant" patients warm almost immediately hearing this. Because it's sometimes the first time they feel like the day in, day out challenge of diabetes has been acknowledged. Do they magically develop normal blood glucose levels? No. But they do often show renewed interest in achieving improved health.

I hope you can use the stories in these pages to open a new conversation, both with your patients and your colleagues. How can we acknowledge these challenges? How can we make things better—is there a way to take just a little of the burden out of the picture? How can we create opportunities for our patients to be partners in care, not just passively receiving lectures and medicines?

I also encourage you to use it as a reminder that every patient is an individual. The American Association of Clinical Endocrinologists encourages us to create individualized goals (and puts out a great diabetes treatment algorithm, by the way). If you have an overweight patient with an A1c of 7.0 percent who can't exercise because they're having low blood sugars, are they better served hanging to that number or by loosening the goal for a while to see if they can lose some weight? The "typical" patient with diabetes may have many atypical challenges that don't show up on a lab sheet.

Finally, if you find this story helpful, encourage your patients to share it with loved ones. Diabetes increases the risk of depression, and some of that may be related to the social isolation of not really knowing how to ask for support. Reading this may be a nice primer for friends and family to have those conversations about how they can form a better network.

We both thank you for listening.

C. Bibliography

"Diabetes." World Health Organization. Accessed December 27, 2016. http://www.who.int/mediacentre/factsheets/fs312/en/.

Fothergill, Erin, Juen Guo, Lilian Howard, Jennifer C. Kerns, Nicolas D. Knuth, Robert Brychta, Kong Y. Chen, Monica C. Skarulis, Mary Walter, Peter J. Walter, and Kevin D. Hall. "Persistent Metabolic Adaptation 6 Years after 'The Biggest Loser' Competition." *Obesity* 24, no. 8 (05, 2016): 1612-619. doi:10.1002/oby.21538.

Levine, Emma Edeman, and Maurice E. Schweitzer. "The Affective and Interpersonal Consequences of Obesity: Weight and the Stereotype Content Model." *SSRN Electronic Journal*. doi:10.2139/ssrn.2258688.

Page, Kathleen A., Owen Chan, Jagriti Arora, Renata Belfort-Deaguiar, James Dzuira, Brian Roehmholdt, Gary W. Cline, Sarita Naik, Rajita Sinha, R. Todd Constable, and Robert S. Sherwin. "Effects of Fructose vs. Glucose on Regional Cerebral Blood Flow in Brain Regions Involved With Appetite and Reward Pathways." *Jama* 309, no. 1 (01, 2013): 63. doi:10.1001/jama.2012.116975.

Stanik-Hutt, Julie, Robin P. Newhouse, Kathleen M. White, Meg Johantgen, Eric B. Bass, George Zangaro, Renee Wilson, Lily Fountain, Donald M. Steinwachs, Lou Heindel, and Jonathan P. Weiner. "The Quality and Effectiveness of Care Provided by Nurse Practitioners." *The Journal for Nurse Practitioners* 9, no. 8 (09 2013). doi:10.1016/j.nurpra.2013.07.004.

Valtorta, Nicole K., Mona Kanaan, Simon Gilbody, Sara Ronzi, and Barbara Hanratty. "Loneliness and Social Isolation as Risk Factors for Coronary Heart Disease and Stroke: Systematic Review and Meta-analysis of Longitudinal Observational Studies." *Heart* 102, no. 13 (04, 2016): 1009-016. doi:10.1136/heartjnl-2015-308790.

www.ingramcontent.com/pod-product-compliance
Lightning Source LLC
Chambersburg PA
CBHW060858280326
41934CB00007B/1099